REDUCING
HIGH BLOOD PRESSURE
FOR BEGINNERS

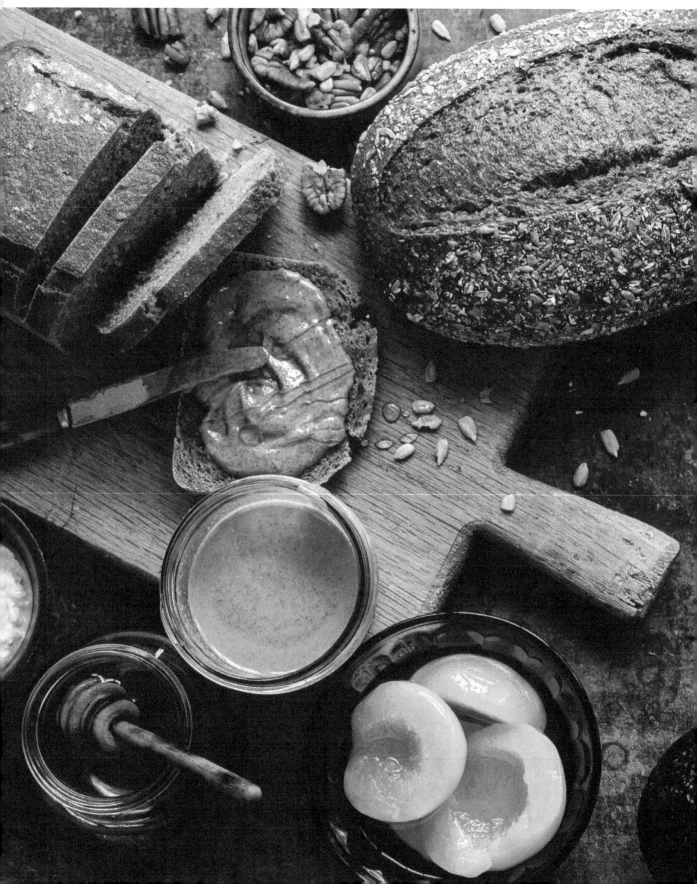

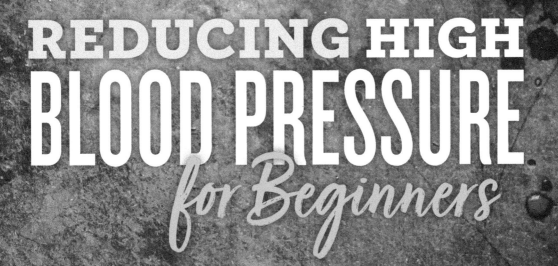

REDUCING HIGH
BLOOD PRESSURE
for Beginners

A COOKBOOK FOR EATING
AND LIVING WELL

KIM LARSON, RDN, NBC-HWC

ROCKRIDGE
PRESS

Interior Designer: Amanda Kirk + Liz Cosgrove
Cover Designer: Liz Cosgrove
Art Producer: Michael Hardgrove
Editor: Lauren O'Neal
Production Editor: Kurt Shulenberger
Photography © 2019 Annie Martin, Food styling by Caroline Franke.
Photography © Nadine Greeff, p. xi; Noelle DeSantis, p. xiii.

ISBN: Print 978-1-64152-880-1 | eBook 978-1-64152-881-8

R0

To my husband, Jim,

who was diagnosed with high blood pressure early in life. Your adventurous culinary palate and drive for better health have helped propel our foodie escapades and our lifelong goal of being active. Thank you for always being ready for the next adventure!

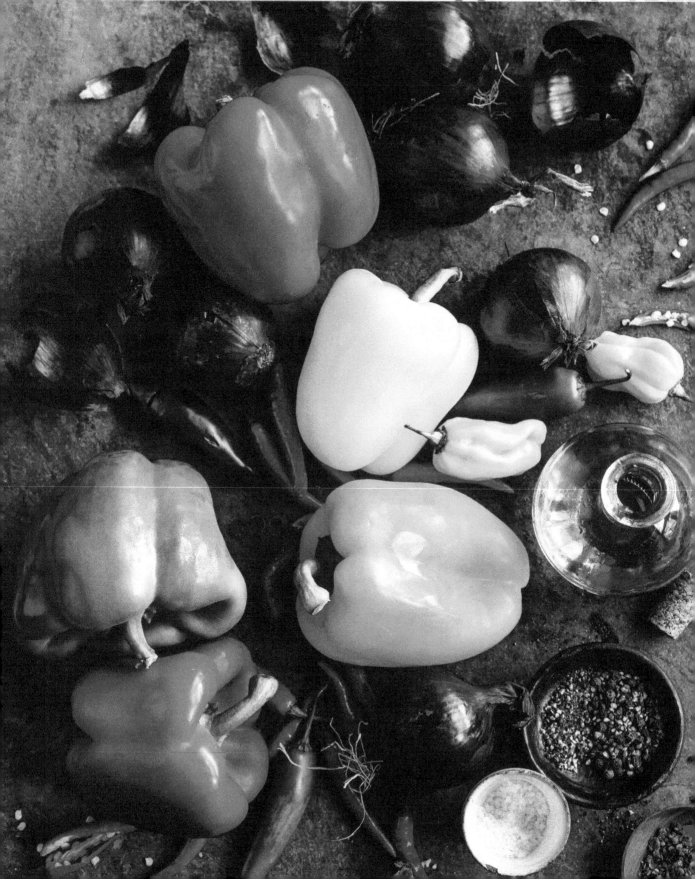

contents

INTRODUCTION

Have you or someone you love been diagnosed with high blood pressure?
If so, you're not alone! In the United States, 46 percent of all adults have high blood pressure, and another 32 percent are at risk of it. High blood pressure is a silent disease: You can have it and not even know it. That means it can be a very surprising diagnosis.

It was surprising for my husband. He was diagnosed with borderline high blood pressure, now called elevated hypertension, during a routine physical exam at 25 years of age. His family history loomed large over this diagnosis because his father died young, at age 46, of a stroke. But because of my husband's healthy diet, exercise, and lifestyle choices since his diagnosis, it wasn't until he was in his forties that he needed to take blood pressure medication—which he's still taking today. His lifestyle choices were, and continue to be, a game changer for his current and future health.

Over the years, we've focused on the daily health habits that bring energy, vitality, and joy to our lives. These include reducing salt intake, making daily exercise a priority, keeping weight control in mind, eating foods that help manage blood pressure, and not smoking. As a registered dietitian nutritionist and certified health and wellness coach, I've helped not only my husband but hundreds of others improve their health by lowering blood pressure with simple changes that make a difference. I'm confident that my book can help you lower your blood pressure, too.

Are you ready to launch your journey to better health? This book contains practical tools, insider knowledge, and delicious recipes to help you reshape your food choices and lifestyle. The first part of this book will outline the whats, whys, and hows of controlling high blood pressure (and heart disease and stroke), with or without medication. The second part is a collection of simple, tasty, and affordable recipes to help ease your transition to a daily diet that supports blood pressure regulation. The journey may be easier than you think!

Healthy nutrition and lifestyle choices are the everyday building blocks for creating a long, healthy, and happy life. Here's to enjoying delicious eating and healthy living—because your life is worth it.

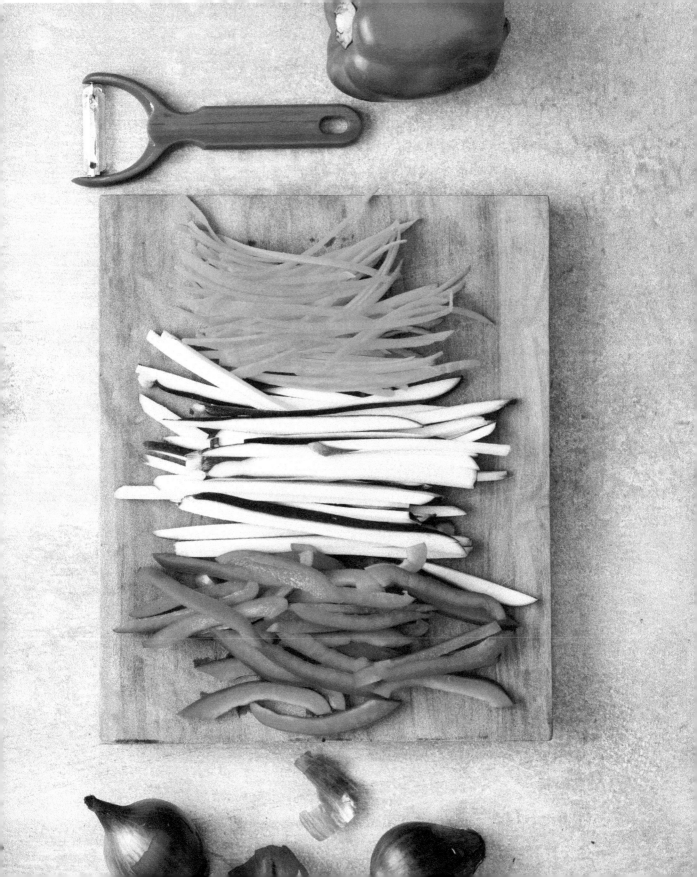

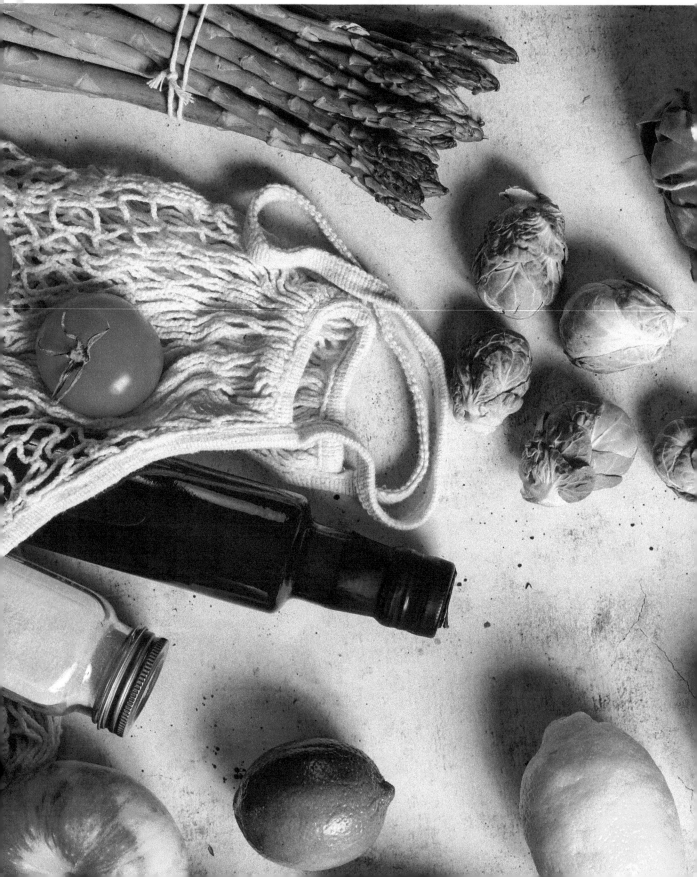

PART ONE
BLOOD PRESSURE 101

Congratulations on beginning the journey to lower your blood pressure! If you want to reduce high blood pressure, making lifestyle changes can be as powerful as taking prescription medications. Isn't that great news? Part 1 of this book will walk you through everything you need to know to take charge of lowering your blood pressure. We'll cover all the essentials, from scientific medical information and healthy living strategies to sample menus and shopping lists. Armed with the best tricks, tips, and tools, you can't help but succeed.

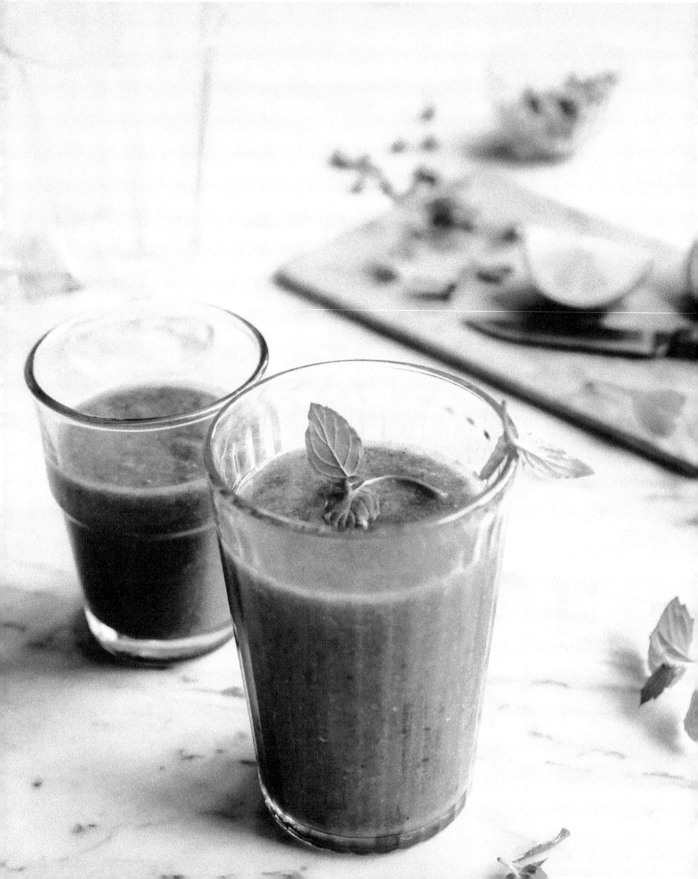

chapter one

SO YOU HAVE HIGH BLOOD PRESSURE

Now that you know you have high blood pressure (also called hypertension), it's time to get started on gaining the knowledge and skills that will help you improve your health. The first step is to understand what high blood pressure is and what it means for your health, both now and in the future. Together we'll explore how to make healthy lifestyle and diet choices a part of your daily routine. Even a small reduction in your blood pressure numbers can improve your lifelong health. The goal is to live your healthiest life—and enjoy every minute of it!

WHAT IS HIGH BLOOD PRESSURE?

As you know, your heart pumps your blood through your arteries and veins. What we call "blood pressure" is the force the blood exerts on the arteries as it's pumped through. We all need a healthy blood pressure to deliver oxygen and nutrients to the cells all over our body. If your blood pressure is too high, it puts a strain on your blood vessels and makes your heart work harder to pump the blood to its destination. This can lead to many negative health consequences. (Your blood pressure shouldn't be too low, either, or you'd faint, but that's not the focus of this book.)

WHAT DOES MY BLOOD PRESSURE READING MEAN?

Your blood pressure reading looks like a fraction, with one number over another, like 120/80 or 140/90. The top number is the systolic pressure, and it measures the pressure of the blood in your arteries *during* heartbeats. The bottom number is the diastolic pressure, and it measures the pressure of the blood in your arteries *between* heartbeats. Blood pressure is measured in millimeters of mercury (mmHg).

On the opposite page are blood pressure classifications by the numbers alongside the categories your healthcare provider will associate with those numbers when discussing them with you.

WHAT CAUSES HIGH BLOOD PRESSURE?

The most common type of high blood pressure is known as essential or primary hypertension. The other type is called secondary hypertension, which is caused by some other medical condition and is much less common. First, let's focus on primary hypertension, which is what people usually mean when they say they've been diagnosed with high blood pressure.

Table 1: **Blood Pressure Classifications**

SYSTOLIC (TOP) NUMBER	DIASTOLIC (BOTTOM) NUMBER	BLOOD PRESSURE CATEGORIES
Less than 120 mmHg	Less than 80 mmHg	Normal (desirable)
120–129 mmHg	Less than 80 mmHg	Elevated
130–139 mmHg	80–89 mmHg	Stage 1 hypertension
140 mmHg or higher	90 mmHg or higher	Stage 2 hypertension
180 mmHg or higher	120 mmHg or higher	Hypertensive crisis

Source: Data adapted from Classification of Blood Pressure, AHA, ACC 2017.

The Causes of Primary Hypertension

High blood pressure can happen at any age—the diagnosis is even becoming more common in infants and children today. In the United States, almost half of all adults now have high blood pressure. Women experience consistent increases after age 55—an increase of 10 mmHg with every decade. Once blood pressure has developed into stage 1 or stage 2 hypertension, it usually lasts a lifetime. There are many different risk factors that contribute to the potential development of high blood pressure. Some you can control; others you can't.

> Caffeine can raise blood pressure, so it's prudent to limit your daily intake to no more than two cups of coffee or two to three servings of other caffeinated beverages such as soda or tea.

Risk Factors You Can't Control

The following issues are the *uncontrollable* factors that influence whether you develop high blood pressure.

Age. According to statistics, about 65 percent of those older than 60 have some form of high blood pressure.

Family history of high blood pressure. There's a genetic tendency for hypertension, so if your parents have it, your chances of developing it are higher.

Gender. Men usually experience high blood pressure earlier in their lives; women are generally protected through menopause.

Race or ethnicity. Black and Latino people have an increased risk of high blood pressure.

Risk Factors You Can Control

These are the main *controllable* lifestyle factors that are known to influence the development of high blood pressure. Even small changes to these factors can have a big effect.

Being overweight or obese. Losing weight (or maintaining your weight) is the first line of defense against high blood pressure, especially as you age.

Physical activity. Regular physical activity can control weight and keep blood pressure stable.

The three S's. Smoking, stress, and sleep apnea have all been found to contribute to high blood pressure.

Drinking alcohol. Regular and heavy alcohol consumption may increase the likelihood of high blood pressure.

Diet, including salt intake. The American Heart Association recommends consuming no more than 2,300 milligrams of salt (sodium) daily to lower blood pressure; if you can lower the amount to 1,500 milligrams daily, even better. (Most Americans consume well over 3,400 milligrams of salt every day.)

The Causes of Secondary Hypertension

About 5 to 10 percent of adults with hypertension have secondary hypertension, meaning it's caused not by diet or lifestyle, but by an already existing medical condition or by the medications or treatments for another condition. There are many different causes of secondary hypertension, including:

- Chemotherapy drugs

- Diabetes

- Disorders associated with low levels of potassium

- Heart or kidney failure
- Herbal supplements such as licorice, ephedra, ginseng, dong quai, and ginkgo
- Hypothyroidism or hyperthyroidism
- Medications such as birth control pills, antidepressants, pain relievers, and decongestants

Even with secondary hypertension, diet and lifestyle changes can make a significant impact alongside the treatments prescribed by your doctor.

COMMON COMORBIDITIES

When someone has two or more disease conditions at the same time, we call those conditions "comorbid." Sometimes the negative health consequences from one disease can make both conditions worse. Examples of conditions that are often comorbid with hypertension include:

- **Coronary artery disease.** High blood pressure contributes to the narrowing and hardening of the coronary arteries. These arteries can clog, leading to a heart attack.

- **Diabetes.** Six of 10 people with diabetes also have high blood pressure, because diabetes can cause changes in our vascular system (the system that pumps blood through our bodies).

- **Kidney disease.** One in five adults with high blood pressure also has kidney disease.

- **Metabolic syndrome.** This diagnosis is given when two or more of these conditions are seen together in one person: high blood pressure, obesity, diabetes, larger waist circumference (greater than 40 inches in men and 35 inches in women), and high blood glucose.

WHAT ARE THE EFFECTS OF HIGH BLOOD PRESSURE?

High blood pressure is dangerous for many reasons. It often causes no symptoms for many years, so you may not even realize you have it. Left unchecked, it can cause permanent damage to blood vessels of the heart, eyes, brain, and kidneys—in fact, high blood pressure is the second leading cause of kidney failure.

It also causes the walls of your arteries to harden and narrow, restricting blood flow and increasing your risk of coronary artery disease and heart attack. Blockages and clots from damage to the arteries can loosen and travel to the brain, causing a stroke. Or the heart could simply wear out and fail, unable to keep up with the body's need to transport blood and oxygen to the organs.

These serious consequences can be avoided by taking effective steps to lower your blood pressure and improve your health with positive and permanent lifestyle changes. That's right: You are in control and can change the path of your health.

WHO HAS HIGH BLOOD PRESSURE?

Now that the American Heart Association's 2017 guidelines have lowered the qualifying criteria, more than half of Americans have high blood pressure. That's a lot! The AHA made this change in part to motivate people to pay attention to their numbers and take action before they reach more advanced stages of hypertension.

The prevalence of high blood pressure varies by people's ethnicity and by where they live, because of genetics and lifestyle and diet choices. According to the Centers for Disease Control, more people in the Southeast and Midwest regions of the United States have high blood pressure. Black and Hispanic adults are also at greater risk. But the truth is people of any age, gender, or race can have high blood pressure.

High blood pressure is very common, so don't feel overwhelmed if you've received this diagnosis. Many of your friends and family likely have high blood pressure of some form or another, just like you. This book will help you start making lifestyle changes that really matter, so you can achieve and maintain a lower, healthier blood pressure level while still enjoying life.

HOW IS HIGH BLOOD PRESSURE TREATED?

There are two main approaches to treating blood pressure: lifestyle changes and medication. It's not an either/or situation; many people use both approaches. Your doctor will help you determine whether medication is necessary, but even if it is, making lifestyle changes is still an effective long-term treatment approach, because it can reduce the amount of medication you need and improve your overall quality of life.

Treating Hypertension with Medication

Medications that your doctor may prescribe to help treat your high blood pressure fall into the following categories:

Alpha blockers cause blood vessels to dilate (open). Examples: terazosin, prazosin (Minipress).

Angiotensin II receptor blockers (ARBs) soften and relax the blood vessels. Examples: candesartan (Atacand), losartan (Cozaar).

Angiotensin-converting enzyme (ACE) inhibitors soften and relax the blood vessels. Examples: lisinopril (Zestril), benazepril (Lotensin), captopril (Capoten).

In the past, treatments for hypertension included bloodletting with leeches, spinal surgery, and injections of typhoid, so we've come a long way! Compared with those archaic approaches, lifestyle changes are easy, enjoyable, manageable, and effective.

Beta blockers lower heart rate and heart contractions. Examples: metoprolol (Lopressor), carvedilol (Coreg), atenolol (Tenormin).

Calcium channel blockers help open the blood vessels so blood can flow more freely. Examples: diltiazem (Cardizem, Tiazac), amlodipine (Norvasc).

Thiazide diuretics, also called "water pills," help the body release water and extra sodium. Example: hydrochlorothiazide (Microzide).

Vasodilators open the blood vessels wider to allow free blood flow. Examples: hydralazine, minoxidil.

Because different drugs lower blood pressure in different ways, your doctor may prescribe more than one drug at a time. Medicine only works if you take it regularly and as your doctor prescribes it, so never stop taking it without consulting your doctor. Also consult with your doctor or registered dietitian nutritionist about foods or other medications that may interact with your blood pressure meds. If you experience side effects like muscle cramps, skin rash, coughing, unusual thirst, constipation, diarrhea, fatigue or drowsiness, insomnia, erectile dysfunction, dizziness or light-headedness, or irregular heartbeat, tell your doctor immediately, but don't stop taking your medications unless directed to by your doctor. It may take a little experimentation to find the right mix of medications for you.

Treating Hypertension the Natural Way

Consistent healthy lifestyle choices, even small ones, have been found to have the biggest effect on every category of high blood pressure. These are the five most important lifestyle steps to take to lower and manage your blood pressure:

1. **Lose weight if you're overweight or obese.** For every 2 pounds of body weight lost, blood pressure drops by 1 mmHg, so losing just 5 percent of your body weight will significantly lower your blood pressure.

2. **Follow the Dietary Approaches to Stop Hypertension (DASH) diet.** Switching to this style of eating has a huge effect on your blood pressure, lowering it

by 8 to 14 mmHg, according to the Preventive Cardiovascular Nurses Association. I'll cover this amazing (and delicious) dietary plan in depth in chapter 2 (page 13).

3. **Lower your daily intake of salt.** You'll see in the next chapter how substitutions and taste boosters can help you avoid salt without sacrificing flavor.

4. **Increase your intake of high-potassium foods** (unless you have kidney disease or take certain medications—check with your doctor first). The specific how-tos of eating more of these foods every day will be discussed in the next chapter.

5. **Don't smoke, and limit alcohol.** If you do smoke, do whatever it takes to stop—permanently.

WEIGHT CONTROL: A VITAL LINK TO BLOOD PRESSURE MANAGEMENT

Maintaining a healthy weight is one of the most significant factors in controlling your blood pressure. The more weight you carry around, the harder your heart and circulatory systems need to work. Excess weight increases your risk of many health problems, including sleep apnea, type 2 diabetes, heart disease, certain cancers, osteoarthritis, and liver and kidney disease, in addition to high blood pressure.

One way to assess your weight is by body mass index (BMI), which is your weight in kilograms divided by the square of your height in meters. The National Institute of Diabetes and Digestive and Kidney Diseases classifies a BMI of 18.5 to 24.9 as normal, 25 to 29.9 as overweight, and 30 or above as obese. Another way to assess your weight is waist size. A waist measurement of 35 inches for women and 40 inches for men elevates your risk of disease. These metrics aren't perfect, but they provide a general idea of healthy weight.

The Power to Treat Your Hypertension

Both medication and lifestyle changes are important treatments for hypertension, but many people choose to control their blood pressure by making healthier lifestyle choices alone rather than going on medication. Why? Because taking a medication is often expensive and not totally risk-free. Drugs can have side effects and long-term downsides that can disrupt your life and distract you from the joy of living far more than any lifestyle changes could. In addition, diet can be just as effective for lowering blood pressure as medicines. Ask your doctor for a referral to a registered dietitian nutritionist to help you with these changes. Even if you do take meds, you'll still benefit from making positive lifestyle changes. Isn't it great to know that you have the power to *take action* to lower your blood pressure? It's never too late (or too early) to protect yourself from hypertension and move confidently toward a healthier, happier, and longer life!

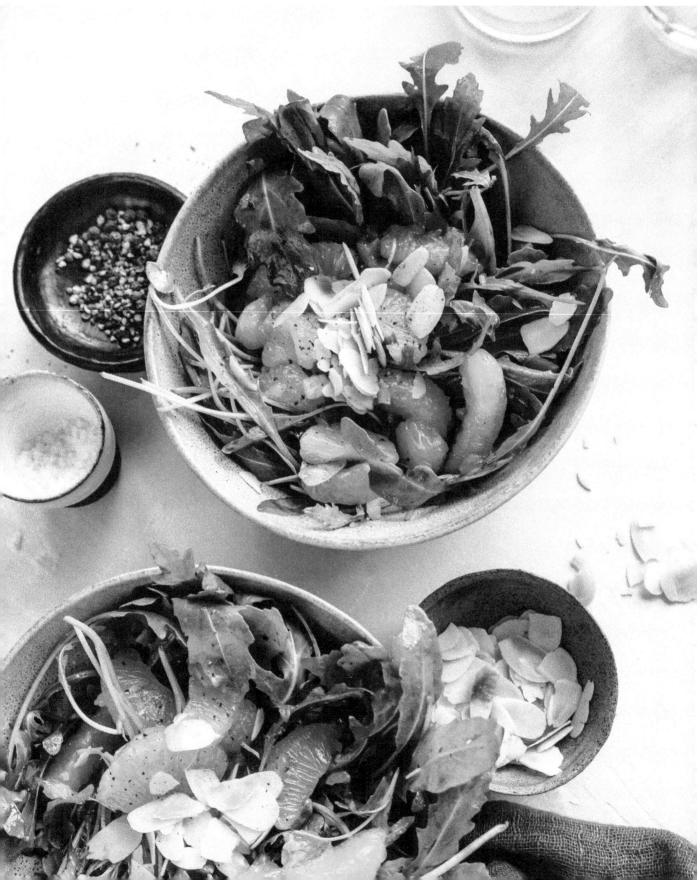

chapter two

LOVING YOUR NEW LIFESTYLE

This chapter provides an overview of how to control your hypertension with food and physical activity. That doesn't mean you have to pay a lot of money for fancy ingredients, spend hours of time in the kitchen preparing meals, or give up enjoying special foods now and then. You can still enjoy the foods you love, with the added bonus of feeling better and being healthier. Your family will enjoy these healthier choices, too!

YOUR NEW WAY OF EATING

What you eat really matters! You may have heard of the DASH diet, or eating a "heart-healthy," "low-salt," or "low-sodium" diet. These are all different ways of describing basically the same thing: eating in a way that controls your blood pressure naturally without medications. For simplicity's sake, I'll refer to this style of eating as the DASH diet. DASH stands for Dietary Approaches to Stop Hypertension. It's an eating plan that's low in salt and saturated fat, and high in fiber, potassium, calcium, and magnesium. Following this plan can help lower your blood pressure in less than a month. In fact, it's been shown to lower blood pressure by 8 to 14 mmHg. All the recipes in this book follow the DASH guidelines, so you can enjoy every recipe with confidence.

In addition to controlling your blood pressure, the DASH diet has many other health benefits. In fact, the *U.S. News & World Report* ranked it in the top five healthiest diets five years running. It lowers low-density lipoprotein (LDL) cholesterol, often called "bad" cholesterol, and it's so well balanced you'll meet most of your nutrition needs without much thought. It may also help you lose weight because it's higher in low-calorie, fiber-rich foods. Many of my clients lose weight on this diet without even trying.

The more closely you follow the diet, the more you'll be surprised at how much better you feel. It has lots of flavor and variety to prevent boredom, and it's so easy to follow. Of course, any kind of change can seem hard at first. As you follow the DASH diet, you'll probably be eating more fruits, vegetables, and whole grains than you're used to. Your taste buds will also need some time to adjust to the lower salt level, but they will. Just start with one or two changes every

Many people control hypertension by eating a vegan or vegetarian diet, but if you're a carnivore, you don't have to give up your favorite meats. You can lower your blood pressure while eating chicken, fish, lean beef, and lean pork. Just add more fruits and vegetables to your plate to achieve your DASH goals.

week and practice those until they become part of your routine. Also, drink lots of water to help your body handle the increase in fiber.

Eat More of These Foods

Restrictive diets are everywhere, but who wants to live like that? Keeping pleasure on your plate is important if you hope to maintain your healthier eating habits. Instead of telling you what you can't eat, the DASH diet encourages you to eat more of the right foods, such as vegetables and fruit, whole grains, lean proteins, nuts and seeds, legumes, and low-fat dairy.

You'll also eat good sources of the minerals calcium, magnesium, and potassium, which are crucial to regulating blood pressure. Be sure to get your potassium, calcium, and magnesium from food sources, not from supplements, because your body doesn't absorb the minerals from supplements as well as from food. Supplements can also interact with other medications, so always check with your doctor before taking any.

Eat Less of These Foods

To make room for more of the essential foods, you'll need to eat less of certain things. These include ultra-processed foods, refined grains and sugars, high-fat dairy products, high-fat meats, alcohol, and high-sodium foods.

One of the most important, but difficult, things to do to control your blood pressure is to reduce your sodium intake. Why is it so important to eat less salt? Salt is "hydrophilic," or attracted to water. When it's present in your bloodstream, it pulls water into your blood vessels, increasing the volume of your blood and thus raising your blood pressure.

Limiting your alcohol intake is recommended by virtually every health organization. Men should have no more than two drinks per day, women no more than one. Sticking with these amounts could lower your blood pressure by 2 to 4 mmHg. Small lifestyle changes can add up to big health benefits!

DAILY DASH

The DASH diet calls for a certain number of daily servings from different food groups. The following table outlines the plan and gives examples of each food and appropriate portion sizes.

FOOD GROUP	SERVINGS PER DAY*	SERVING SIZES	EXAMPLES AND NOTES	SIGNIFICANCE OF EACH FOOD GROUP TO THE DASH DIET
Whole grains	6 to 8	1 slice bread 1 ounce dry cereal ½ cup cooked rice, pasta, or cereal	Whole-wheat bagels, bread, pasta, and pitas; cereal; grits; oatmeal; brown rice; unsalted popcorn	Major sources of energy and fiber
Vegetables	4 to 5	1 cup raw leafy vegetables ½ cup cut-up raw or cooked vegetables ½ cup vegetable juice	Broccoli, carrots, collard greens, green beans, green peas, kale, lima beans, potatoes, spinach, squash, sweet potatoes, tomatoes	Rich sources of potassium, magnesium, and fiber
Fruits	4 to 5	1 medium fruit ¼ cup dried fruit ½ cup fresh, frozen, or canned fruit ½ cup fruit juice	Apples, apricots, bananas, dates, grapefruit, grapes, oranges, mangos, melons, peaches, pineapples, raisins, strawberries, tangerines	Important sources of potassium, magnesium, and fiber
Fat-free/ low-fat dairy	2 to 3	1 cup milk or yogurt 1½ ounces cheese	Fat-free (skim) or low-fat (1%) milk or buttermilk; fat-free, low-fat, or reduced-fat cheese; fat-free or low-fat regular or frozen yogurt	Major sources of calcium and protein

*for a 2000-calorie diet

FOOD GROUP	SERVINGS PER DAY*	SERVING SIZES	EXAMPLES AND NOTES	SIGNIFICANCE OF EACH FOOD GROUP TO THE DASH DIET
Lean meats, poultry, and fish	6 or fewer	1 ounce cooked meat, poultry, or fish 1 egg (no more than 4 yolks per week)	Select only lean meats; trim away visible fat; broil, roast, or poach; remove skin from poultry	Rich sources of protein and magnesium
Nuts, seeds, and legumes	4 to 5 per week	⅓ cup or 1½ ounces nuts 2 tablespoons peanut butter 2 tablespoons or ½ ounce seeds ½ cup cooked legumes (beans/peas)	Almonds, hazelnuts, mixed nuts, peanut butter, peanuts, walnuts, sunflower seeds, kidney beans, lentils, split peas	Rich sources of energy, magnesium, protein, and fiber
Fats and oils	2 to 3	1 teaspoon soft margarine 1 teaspoon vegetable oil 1 tablespoon mayonnaise 2 tablespoons salad dressing	Soft margarine, vegetable oils (canola, corn, olive, safflower), low-fat mayonnaise, light salad dressing	About 27% of calories on the DASH diet come from fat
Sweets and added sugars	5 or fewer per week	1 tablespoon sugar 1 tablespoon jelly or jam ½ cup sorbet or gelatin 1 cup lemonade	Fruit-flavored gelatin, fruit punch, hard candy, jelly, maple syrup, sorbet and ices, sugar	Sweets should be low in fat

Source: Adapted from *Your Guide to Lowering Your Blood Pressure with DASH*, U.S. Department of Health and Human Services, National Institutes of Health, National Heart, Lung, and Blood Institute.

Most of us consume too much salt without even realizing it—more than 3,400 milligrams (mg) of sodium per day on average. The American Heart Association recommends no more than 2,300 mg of sodium (1 teaspoon of salt) per day. An even lower amount, 1,500 mg per day (less than 0.75 teaspoons salt), is recommended for adults older than 50, African Americans, and people with high blood pressure. According to research, eating less than 2,300 mg of salt a day can lower blood pressure by 2 to 8 mmHg. Even cutting back by 1,000 mg per day can significantly improve your blood pressure numbers.

About 70 percent of the sodium we eat comes from processed foods like boxed, prepared, or packaged foods. You can easily lower your salt intake by eating more whole foods like fresh fruits and vegetables, but you can still eat frozen or canned produce if you check the labels for salt and sugar first. Rinsing canned food can also reduce salt by up to 40 percent.

EATING AT A RESTAURANT

Your days of eating out at restaurants are not over! You just have to know how to make healthier decisions when you're out. Learn to politely but assertively ask the waitstaff for what you need; most restaurants are very accommodating.

How to Order

Here are some steps to take to eat healthy when you eat out:

- Ask for water, regular coffee, zero-calorie tea, or low-fat milk.

- Ask how sides like potatoes and cooked vegetables are prepared, and request that they be steamed and served plain, if necessary.

- Choose entrées that come with a vegetable.

- Request an additional vegetable or a salad (with dressing on the side) to accompany your meal or to replace a less-healthy side dish (such as French fries).

- Select foods prepared with herbs, spices, citrus juices, or vinegars.

- Select foods that are broiled, baked, grilled, or braised in their own juices.

What Not to Order

Here are foods to avoid when eating out:

- All fast food, such as pizza, burgers, and hot dogs

- Broth-based entrées or soups

- Condiments such as ketchup, mustard, or gravy

- Dishes with a lot of cheese (either regular or processed)

- Foods prepared with monosodium glutamate (MSG) or seasoning salts

- Foods that are fried, deep-fried, sautéed, and/or breaded

- Foods that are pickled, cured, or smoked

- Processed meats such as bacon, ham, sausages, deli meats, and jerky

- Salty foods such as olives, pickles, tomato juice, canned meats, and sauerkraut

- Sauces such as barbecue, Worcestershire, soy, tartar, and teriyaki

- Soda, juice, and alcohol

IN THE GROCERY STORE

Surrounding yourself with the foods you enjoy makes it easier to stick with your new way of eating. Here are some shopping tips to help you keep your kitchen stocked with tasty and nutritious foods:

- Choose fresh or frozen vegetables (without added sugar or salt).

- Choose fresh, freeze-dried, or dried herbs to flavor foods.

- Choose low-salt or reduced-sodium versions of canned broth, soup, tuna, tomatoes, beans, and other vegetables.

- Choose low-salt versions of crackers, bread, and cereal.

- Choose lower-sodium boxed cereals.

- Look at your grocery cart before checking out: Is one-third of it filled with produce (fresh, frozen, or canned)?

- Look for salt-free seasoning blends (e.g., Mrs. Dash) in the spice section.

- Look for sauces with no salt, or avoid prepared sauces and make your own (see chapter 10, page 157).

- Plan your meals and bring your shopping list of recipe ingredients, staples, and perishables.

- Read the labels on salad dressings; consider making your own (see chapter 10, page 157).

- Skip boxed rice and pasta mixes.

- Skip deli and processed meats; use fresh instead.

- Skip frozen meals and pizzas, which are high in sodium.

- Skip pickles, olives, and condiments high in sodium.

- Skip quick-cooking foods, especially cereals such as instant oatmeal.

- Try Lundberg Whole Grain Rice Mixes, which contain no added salt.

HEALTHY SNACKS

Snacking on healthy foods is a great way to boost your nutrition. You don't have to stop snacking when you follow the DASH plan; just surround yourself with snacks that are low in sodium but high in nutrients (particularly potassium and calcium). Here are a few of my favorites:

- Fresh fruit
- Fresh raw veggies
- Frozen blueberries, grapes, or bananas
- Homemade trail mix of unsalted nuts, seeds, and dried fruit
- Low-fat plain Greek yogurt with fresh or frozen fruit
- Low-salt or no-salt popcorn
- Low-salt tomato or V-8 juice
- Low-salt tuna with low-fat cottage cheese
- Unsalted nuts

Label Lingo

Read the labels on packaged foods. If salt is in the top three ingredients on the ingredients list, avoid it. Keep in mind that you should also look out for the words *brined, marinated, smoked, baking soda, sea salt, salt flakes, savory, NaCl* (sodium chloride), and *seasoned*.

The Nutrition Facts panel on the package lists the total amount of sodium, in milligrams and as a percentage of the daily recommended value. Choose foods that contain less than 5 percent of the daily recommended value of sodium and avoid foods with 20 percent or more. (Remember, you're aiming for a total of 2,300 milligrams of sodium or less per day—or 1,500 milligrams if your doctor has recommended it.)

What about phrases like "no salt added" or "reduced sodium" on food labels? Here's a guide to those claims and what they mean:

Table 2: **Salt Claims on Products**

CLAIM	WHAT IT MEANS
No salt added; unsalted	No salt added during processing (not a sodium-free food)
Light in sodium	50 percent less sodium than the regular version
Reduced or lower sodium	At least 25 percent less sodium than the regular version
Low-sodium meal	140 mg or less sodium per 3.5 ounces (100 grams)
Low-sodium	140 mg or less sodium per serving
Very low sodium	35 mg or less sodium per serving
Sodium-free or salt-free	Less than 5 mg sodium per serving

Source: *Your Guide to Lowering Your Blood Pressure with DASH*, U.S. Department of Health and Human Services, National Institutes of Health, National Heart, Lung, and Blood Institute, Table 11.

EXERCISE MADE EASY

Studies show that daily movement or exercise helps bring your blood pressure down and keep it down. That means that getting in some form of physical activity should become a habit for you, like brushing your teeth every day. Exercising, or even just moving your body more, can seem daunting if you're not used to it, but it doesn't have to be. You can make simple changes in your life that will nudge you into a more active style of living one day at a time. For example, it's surprisingly easy to take more steps throughout the day.

Fitting Fitness into Your Day

Here are some ways to enjoy moving more throughout your day—and perhaps even checking some items off your to-do list along the way:

- Ask a friend or family member to join you on a walk or jog.

- Explore nature on a hike.

- Go dancing.

- Join a gym.

- Park your car farther away from the store when you run errands.

- Ride your bike or walk when you visit a friend or run errands nearby.

- Take the stairs wherever you go; avoid elevators.

- Try a yoga class.

- Walk for 10 minutes before work, during your lunch hour, and when you get home from work.

- Walk in a mall when the weather is bad.

- Walk or run around the field while waiting for your children's sports practice to end.

- Walk your dog, or volunteer to walk dogs at a nearby shelter.

Walk It Out

How do you start a regular exercise routine? If you've been sedentary for a while, I recommend starting with walking. It's an easy way to get up and go without needing a gym membership or any equipment, and you can make good progress by gradually adding speed, time, and resistance to get more fit.

Start with just 10 minutes a day on three days each week, walking at a comfortable speed—not slow, but not fast, either. After doing that for a week or two, add another 10-minute walking session and do two walks a day for another few weeks. Finally, add a final 10-minute session, repeating the previous steps. Any combination of walk time is fine, as long as you get in a total of 30 minutes each day.

Keep that schedule for at least four weeks until it's a comfortable part of your weekly routine. When you're ready, add those walks to two more days, on the weekend or during the week, so that you're walking for 30 minutes a day, five times a week. Next, increase your speed to a brisk pace (about 3.5 miles per hour). You are now meeting the minimum time recommended for daily physical activity by the American College of Sports Medicine (ACSM): 30 minutes a day, five days a week, or 2.5 hours a week. This amount of exercise can lower your blood pressure by 4 to 9 mmHg. If losing weight is one of your goals, you'll need to keep increasing the walking time.

Keep this walking regimen up by inviting a friend, coworker, or partner to join you. Walk and talk!

Aerobic Exercise

Aerobic exercise, also known as "cardio," is the kind of exercise that gets your heart pumping, so you can see why it's important for heart health. The ACSM recommends getting 150 minutes of moderate aerobic exercise or 75 minutes of vigorous aerobic exercise per week.

Brisk walking is a convenient choice for moderate aerobic exercise, but you could also try jogging, raking leaves, shoveling snow, climbing stairs, gardening,

Important note: Check with your doctor before beginning any type of exercise program to be sure you're able to proceed. Some people with high blood pressure need to take extra precautions.

mowing the lawn, water aerobics, or bicycling. For vigorous exercise, try things like jumping rope, walking on an incline, singles tennis, bicycling uphill, or swimming laps.

The more exercise you do regularly, the more health benefits you will reap! Studies demonstrate that being consistent with your physical activity and doing more of it is better for health than sporadic bouts, but any kind of exercise is a step in the right direction.

Strength Training

In addition to aerobic exercise, the ACSM recommends including two sessions of strength training, also known as resistance training or weight training, every week. Whereas aerobic exercise focuses on your heart and lungs, strength training focuses on your muscles. It can be done with dumbbells, barbells, bands, kettlebells, or your own bodyweight—anything that has weight will work. You don't need to be inside a gym or use special equipment. Lifting gallons of milk or even soup cans can build muscle when you're first starting out!

Strength training has metabolic benefits that reach far beyond building and maintaining muscle strength. It helps your body more efficiently use the insulin your pancreas secretes, which keeps your blood sugar in a healthy range. It also helps you burn more calories because muscle burns more calories than fat tissue. That benefit helps us manage our weight better over the long term by keeping our level of body fat within a reasonable range.

Sleep affects our moods, energy, and hormone levels; improves our ability to maintain a healthy weight; and boosts overall quality of life. Aim for a minimum of seven to nine hours of quality sleep nightly.

DE-STRESS FOR SUCCESS

We all have stress in our lives, but when stress mounts, it can wreak havoc on your mental and physical health. (Just think about how you can almost feel your blood pressure rising when you're in a frustrating situation.) Fortunately, there are things you can do to help manage stress so it doesn't contribute to your high blood pressure. Consider trying one or more of these coping strategies to help lower your daily stress:

- Create more "down" time to recharge.
- Listen to music.
- Meditate.
- Perform daily physical activity.
- Pray.
- Use relaxation techniques such as mindfulness and deep breathing.
- Spend time with friends and family.
- Start a gratitude or mindfulness journal.
- Take up tai chi.
- Talk to a friend or therapist.
- Volunteer to help others.

As with diet and exercise, don't expect results overnight. The important thing is to address your stress level and begin to change how you handle it. It will make a difference in your life and your health.

YOU CAN DO IT!

The first step to changing your life forever is learning about how your lifestyle affects your blood pressure and deciding to do something about it. These first two chapters have given you the information and understanding that will guide you on your way to controlling your blood pressure and lifestyle choices. The next chapter will give you useful tools and practical steps for your journey to a healthier lifestyle. I'm excited to share them with you!

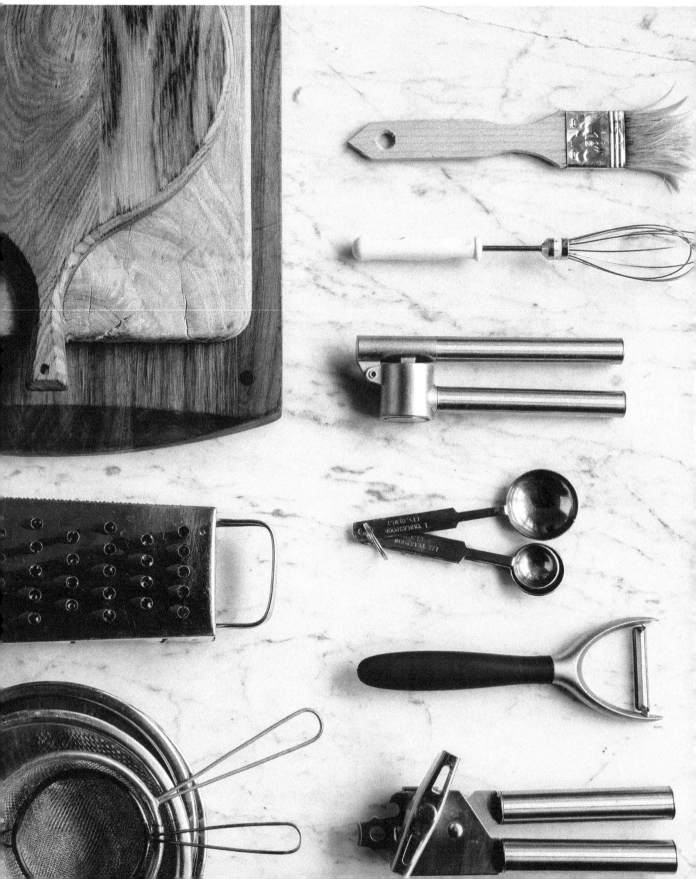

chapter three

EVERYTHING YOU NEED TO MASTER YOUR HEALTH

With a few simple lifestyle changes, you'll soon be reaping the benefits of lower blood pressure and better overall health. Taking control of your health will help you build the confidence and skills you need for a lifetime of wellness. This chapter will make the process even easier by giving you the details of your new eating plan, from cooking tips to product suggestions—even a sample grocery list and menu. These practical tools will elevate your enjoyment of eating without sacrificing ease, accessibility, or budget.

STOCKING YOUR KITCHEN

Making delicious meals doesn't have to be complicated. I believe time in the kitchen should be productive, efficient, and fun! That's easier to do if you have everything you need. Here are a few pieces of kitchen equipment to help you create the healthy foods in this book.

Must-Have Equipment

Here's a list of the equipment I consider most important for making the recipes in this book:

Baking sheet with ½-inch rim.

Blender.

Box grater. This multifunction tool can grate, shave, zest, slice, and shred, depending on which side you use.

Can opener. Canned foods are convenient and budget friendly, so get a good can opener that's easy to use and cleans well in the dishwasher.

Colander and sieve.

Cutting boards. Choose wood or a hard plastic that doesn't stain or absorb flavors. You'll want to have a few, in different sizes.

Large whisk and small whisk.

Measuring spoons and measuring cups.

Multi-size mixing bowls. I prefer stainless steel bowls because they don't affect the taste of the food and they can take a lot of beating in the kitchen.

Sets of pots and pans. I like nonstick pots and pans for easy cleanup and care. Buy a moderately priced set that includes at least one stockpot or Dutch oven, a few smaller pots and pans, a skillet or frying pan, and a sauté pan (deeper than a frying pan, with straight sides).

Sharp knives of different sizes and a good knife sharpener.

A silicone brush or two. This small kitchen tool will save you lots of calories by evenly distributing a small amount of oil for cooking (yes, you can use less oil if you have this brush!).

Vegetable peeler.

Nice-to-Have Equipment

Here's a list of cookware items that aren't necessary for preparing the recipes in this book but would facilitate preparation:

Food chopper. Mine is from Pampered Chef, and the blades stay sharp.

Food processor. This is a luxury kitchen item but worth the money if you like to cook from scratch, use recipes with lots of ingredients, or entertain large groups.

Grill pan. These pans cook single pieces of meat in a flash and leave those wonderful grill marks that make food look especially appealing.

Juicer or lemon press.

Salad spinner.

Slow cooker.

Tongs.

Microplane or zester. Because citrus zest adds so much flavor to dishes in the absence of salt, a sharp and ergonomically friendly zester is a good tool to have.

Build a healthier plate by visualizing your plate divided into fourths. Fill two quarters with vegetables, one with protein, and one with whole grains. Dishes with a mix of several food groups are great to include!

STOCKING YOUR PANTRY

A well-stocked pantry is the key to easy, delicious, and healthy eating. It's also a huge time-saver! Having standard ingredients at your fingertips removes the hassle of having to go out to the grocery store for every recipe you make. These are basics that you should have on hand. This list is not all-inclusive—it's just a place to start when making the recipes in this book. To go easy on the budget, don't buy everything at once.

Dried fruit. Sun-dried tomatoes, cranberries, raisins, apricots, or other dried fruit to add to recipes or eat as a snack.

Dried legumes. You can purchase bags of lentils, peas, and beans, if you prefer to cook them from scratch rather than buy canned.

Extra-virgin olive oil (EVOO), canola oil, and avocado oil. EVOO is great for lower stove temperatures, canola oil for medium-high heat, and avocado oil for high-temperature cooking such as stir-frying.

Low-salt baking powder and baking soda.

Nuts and seeds. Nuts should be either dry-roasted or raw, and either unsalted or with reduced salt. I recommend almonds, walnuts, pistachios, pumpkin seeds (shelled), sunflower seeds (shelled), chia seeds, and sesame seeds.

Old-fashioned rolled oats.

Reduced-sodium canned foods. Tomatoes, tomato sauce or paste, beans, broth, tuna, and corn all fit the bill.

Consuming two to three servings of low-fat dairy every day is an important piece of the DASH diet. Dairy products contain nutrients that lower blood pressure, e.g., potassium, calcium, magnesium, and phosphorus. Gradually increase your dairy consumption by swapping out sweetened tea or soda for low-fat milk at mealtimes.

Spices. Reducing your salt intake doesn't mean you have to eat bland food! Recipes in this book call for dried herbs and spices such as basil, thyme, oregano, rosemary, ginger, paprika, chili powder, cumin, cayenne pepper, and red pepper flakes. I also recommend garlic and onion powder (not garlic salt or onion salt). My favorite salt-free dried spice brands include Mrs. Dash, The Spice House, Litehouse, and McCormick's Perfect Pinch.

Vinegars. The recipes in this book use balsamic, apple-cider, white, white-wine, and red-wine vinegars.

Whole grains. Brown rice and quinoa are particularly useful for the recipes in this book.

Flour and whole-wheat pastry flour.

Whole-wheat pasta and whole-wheat bread. Bean-based pastas (such as Banza) are also good choices if you eat gluten-free.

TIPS AND TRICKS

The following tips and tricks will accelerate your transition to this new eating style and help you avoid some pitfalls:

- **After chopping garlic, let it sit for 10 to 15 minutes before using it.** This lets health-promoting enzymes activate so you can reap the full health benefits.

- **Don't add salt to cooking water, even when it's called for (often in cooking instructions of pasta, rice, or other whole grains).** When broth is called for, use water.

- **Hide the salt shaker and begin to taste your food in a new way.** If you really need to punch up the flavor, try adding a sprinkle of an herb or spice, or a splash of lemon.

- **If your meal includes a vegetable, double or triple it.** You can increase the amount of the same vegetable or add others. That will increase your nutrient intake and automatically lower the salt content because you're increasing the volume of the dish.

- **If you're a big meat eater, cut your meat portions by a half or a third at each meal.**

- **Make a habit of planning your meals on Sundays for the following week.**

- **Make one or two changes in your food choices at a time.** Don't try to do everything all at once.

- **Once a week, "batch-cook" a recipe, doubling or tripling it so you'll have extra to eat as leftovers or freeze for later.**

- **Rinse canned foods (even low-sodium ones) such as beans or corn before using them, to remove some of the sodium.**

- **Use leftovers to create a new meal and avoid wasting food.** You'll find examples of how to repurpose leftovers in a few recipes in this book.

- **When making your favorite recipes, cut the salt in half.** After several months, you may be able to skip it altogether. (Note: This tip does not work in baking because salt controls fermentation in breads and is used as a tenderizer, flavor enhancer, and preservative in other baked goods.)

- **When you've lowered your salt intake consistently, you'll notice a dramatic difference in salt intensity when you taste foods that are high in salt.** We become more sensitized to salt when we eat less of it. The same goes for sugar.

- **Be patient and trust the process detailed in this book.** You'll achieve the results you want in time!

WHAT TO EAT THIS WEEK

To help you get started, I've put together a one-week sample menu (and a grocery list to go with it). This menu is not a calorie-controlled pattern for weight loss, but rather an example of what DASH-focused daily meals might be like for one week, using some of the recipes in this book. Adjust the portions to meet your individual daily calorie needs. If you need help determining what those are, contact a registered dietitian nutritionist near you.

All ingredients needed for the recipes for the week are included on the grocery list, but be sure to check your pantry and refrigerator before you head to the store—you probably already have some common staples and spices. The out-of-the-ordinary ingredients are on this list so you can try them. Substitute different fresh, frozen, or canned produce as you see fit to make these meals your own. Of course, you may not want to follow the meal plan exactly, so feel free to make your own shopping list that only uses ingredients for the recipes you want to make.

One-Week Grocery List

Dairy

1½ gallons nonfat or low-fat milk

1 pint half-and-half

1 (8-ounce) carton nonfat plain
Greek yogurt

1 small carton crumbled blue cheese

1 small carton crumbled goat cheese

1 small carton crumbled low-sodium
feta cheese

1 small (8-ounce) carton light sour cream

1 (16-ounce) tub low-fat cottage cheese

Breads, Cereals, Boxed Items

1 loaf whole-wheat bread

1 (42-ounce) box old-fashioned oats

4 whole-grain or whole-wheat rolls

1 (16-ounce) bag Lundberg Wild Rice
Pilaf Mix

1 (16.4-ounce) box shredded
wheat cereal

1 (16-ounce) box whole-wheat couscous

1 (32-ounce) bag brown rice

1 box Nature's Path Honey Almond Granola
(or another low-sodium cereal such as Kashi
Heart to Heart)

1 bag tricolor quinoa

1 box bulgur

Canned Items

4 (15.5-ounce) cans low-sodium chickpeas

2 (15.5-ounce) cans low-sodium great
northern beans

1 (15.5-ounce) can low-sodium
cannellini beans

2 (14.5-ounce) cans diced tomatoes (no
salt added)

1 (8-ounce) can tomato sauce (no
salt added)

1 (14.5-ounce) can crushed tomatoes (no
salt added)

1 (6-ounce) can tomato paste (no
salt added)

2 (14.5 ounce) cans low-sodium whole
tomatoes

1 (12-ounce) bottle low-sodium V-8 or
tomato juice

1 (4-ounce) can diced green chiles

1 (12-ounce) can pineapple slices,
in pineapple juice

1 (12-ounce) can evaporated milk

1 small bottle/can apricot juice/nectar,
no sugar added

1 (12-ounce) can diced mangos, in their
own juice

1 (14-ounce) can artichokes

2 (13.5-ounce) cans unsweetened light
coconut milk

1 (10-ounce) can mandarin oranges, in their
own juice

2 (14.5-ounce) cans low-sodium
vegetable broth

2 (14.5-ounce) cans low-sodium
chicken broth

1 (16-ounce) jar low-salt peanut butter

1 (16-ounce) jar low-salt almond butter

Cooking, Baking

1 (8-ounce) bag whole-wheat panko bread crumbs

1 (24-ounce) bottle canola oil

1 (16-ounce) bottle extra-virgin olive oil

1 (5-ounce) bottle toasted sesame oil

1 (12-ounce) bottle honey

1 (2.5-ounce) bottle Mrs. Dash No-Salt Lemon Pepper Seasoning

1 (8-ounce) bag unsweetened shredded coconut

1 (8-ounce) bag toffee bits

1 (12-ounce) bag semisweet chocolate chips

1 (12-ounce) bottle balsamic vinegar

1 (12-ounce) bottle white balsamic vinegar

1 (12.7-ounce) bottle white-wine vinegar

1 (12.7-ounce) bottle red-wine vinegar

1 (5-ounce) bag reduced-sugar dried cranberries

1 (3-pound) bag whole-wheat pastry flour

12 standard-size paper muffin liners

1 (1-ounce) bottle vanilla extract

1 (1.7-ounce) bottle pure maple syrup

1 (8-ounce) jar whole-grain mustard

1 (8-ounce) jar Dijon mustard

1 (2.5-ounce) jar Jane's Krazy Original Mixed-Up Pepper

1 (12-ounce) bottle sweet chili sauce

1 (16-ounce) bottle apple-cider vinegar

Nuts, Seeds, Dried Fruit

1 (1-pound) bag unsalted raw pecans

2 cups unsalted raw shelled sunflower seeds

1 cup unsalted chopped raw walnuts

1 cup unsalted toasted almonds

1 cup unsalted raw shelled pumpkin seeds

1 (8-ounce) bag dried apricots

1 (10-ounce) bag golden raisins

Herbs

2 large bunches fresh basil

1 package fresh chives

1 bunch fresh parsley

1 bunch fresh cilantro (optional)

1 package fresh thyme

1 package fresh rosemary

Meats, Poultry, Fish, Eggs, Seafood

1 dozen eggs

10 to 12 skinless, boneless chicken thighs

4 split chicken breasts

1- to 2-pound bag frozen raw wild shrimp (21–30 count)

2 pounds halibut fillet (or cod, tilapia, black cod, or rockfish)

4 sirloin tip steaks

1.5 pounds beef tri-tip strips

1 pound boneless, skinless chicken breasts

1 pound beef stew meat

4 thick-cut boneless pork loins

Vegetables, Fruit

1 apple

3 heads garlic

1 bag/head romaine

16 ounces strawberries

2 medium crowns broccoli

3 kiwis

3 fresh limes

3 lemons

¾ pound green beans

1 small bunch lacinato (black) kale

1 small bag baby carrots

1 (2-pound) bag carrots

2 small bags grated carrots

2 heads celery

1 (5-pound) bag russet potatoes

1 small bag baby red potatoes

1 small bag fingerling or bite-sized potatoes

1 bag spring mix greens

12 large shallots

4 red bell peppers

1 (7-ounce) bag arugula

1 medium yellow onion

1 small butternut squash (or 2 cups precut cubes)

12 ounces apple juice (no sugar added)

1 large white onion

1 (10-ounce) bag mixed broccoli and cauliflower florets

2 small zucchini

2 (8-ounce) packages mushrooms

1 (8-ounce) package cherry tomatoes

2 pounds fresh tomatoes

2 bunches green onions

3 red onions

2 sweet onions

5 (6-ounce) bags baby spinach

1 cantaloupe

3 bananas

1 small bag snap-pea pods

Frozen Vegetables, Fruit, Fruit Juices

2 small bags frozen blueberries

1 bag frozen peaches

1 (6-ounce) can orange juice concentrate (no sugar added)

1 (14.4-ounce) bag pearl onions

1 (12-ounce) bag green peas

ONE-WEEK MEAL PLAN

MEAL	DAY 1	DAY 2	DAY 3
Breakfast	Orange-Berry Swirl (page 49) Whole-wheat toast or English muffin with low-salt peanut butter	4 ounces low-salt V-8 or low-salt tomato juice Low-fat or nonfat Greek yogurt (plain or flavored) Homemade Muesli (page 43) (with yogurt parfait or low-fat or nonfat milk)	Cooked oatmeal with unsalted almond slices and diced mangos (frozen or canned in own juice) Whole-wheat toast with low-fat/low-salt margarine 6 ounces orange juice
Lunch	Moroccan Kale and Bulgur Salad (page 58) Apple slices with nonfat plain Greek yogurt or low-fat vanilla yogurt, sprinkled with cinnamon 8 ounces low-fat or nonfat milk	Butternut Squash and Cannellini Bean Soup (page 70) Mandarin Orange, Arugula, and Almond Salad (page 68) Fresh seasonal fruit 8 ounces low-fat or skim milk	Fireside Beef Stew (page 56) Raw veggies with Spinach and Chickpea Dip (page 147) Whole-grain roll Frozen sliced peaches (no added sugar), thawed 8 ounces low-fat or nonfat milk
Afternoon Snack	Carrot and celery sticks	Cottage Cheese, Chive, and Tomato Salad (page 148)	Mixed berries
Dinner	Grilled Steak with Roasted Onions and Peppers (page 122) Mashed potatoes (no salt) Steamed spinach with splash of lemon juice Sliced tomato salad with drizzle of balsamic vinegar and olive oil, sprinkled with fresh chopped basil Fresh cantaloupe, diced 8 ounces low-fat or skim milk	Spicy Chickpeas over Rice (page 81) Sensational Sautéed Greens (page 67) Strawberries with Honey-Cream Topping (page 153) 8 ounces low-fat or nonfat milk	Pork Loins with Velvety Whole-Grain Mustard Sauce (page 142) Garlic Roasted Red Potatoes (page 64) Charred Stovetop Broccoli (page 65) Spring Greens with Apricots, Goat Cheese, and Sizzled Shallots (page 61) with Everyday Herb Vinaigrette (page 163) 8 ounces low-fat or nonfat milk

DAY 4	DAY 5	DAY 6	DAY 7
Apricot nectar (no added sugar) Blueberry Oat Muffin (page 46) Hardboiled egg	6 ounces low-salt V-8 or low-salt tomato juice Bran flakes with sliced banana and low-fat or nonfat milk	Orange sections Nutty Banana Toast (page 44)	6 ounces orange juice Everything Egg Scramble (page 42) Whole-wheat English muffin Kiwi-and-blueberry fruit bowl
Citrus Shrimp and Spinach Salad (page 62) Whole-wheat roll 8 ounces low-fat or nonfat milk	Mediterranean Quinoa Salad (page 60) served over arugula Fruit (fresh, frozen, or canned in its own juices, no sugar) 8 ounces low-fat or nonfat milk	Braised White Beans with Spinach (page 80) Low-fat or nonfat milk Fruit (fresh, frozen, or canned in its own juices, no sugar)	Chicken Curry in a Hurry (page 106) Low-fat or nonfat Greek yogurt, flavored or plain
Fruit (fresh, frozen, or canned in its own juices, no sugar)	Spiced Honey-Roasted Pecans (page 149)	Fresh fruit	Trail mix
Lemon-Pepper Baked Chicken (page 117) Baked potato with nonfat Greek yogurt and chopped chives Romaine garden salad 8 ounces low-fat or nonfat milk	Sweet-and-Savory Chicken over Couscous (page 114) Roasted cauliflower Grilled Pineapple with Maple-Pecan Drizzle (page 152) 8 ounces low-fat or nonfat milk	Halibut with Roasted Tomato and Basil Sauce (page 107) and Lundberg Wild Rice Pilaf Steamed green beans Chocolate-Coconut Pots de Crème (page 150) 8 ounces low-fat or nonfat milk	Balsamic Beef-and-Vegetable Kebabs (page 134) over brown rice 8 ounces low-fat or nonfat milk

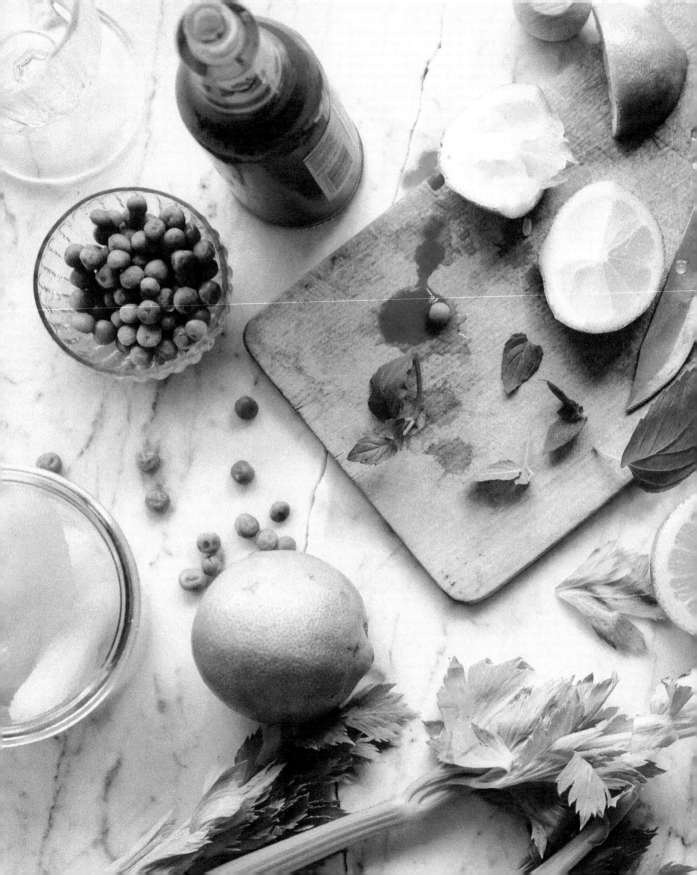

PART TWO

RECIPES FOR EATING AND LIVING WELL

This part of the book gives you simple, tasty, blood pressure–friendly meals you can feel good about making and eating. The recipes are designed to be easy, quick, inexpensive, low in salt, and full of flavor. None of the recipes use salt substitutes, which can interact with some medications. On each recipe, you'll see one or more of the following labels:

1 Pot: Uses only one cooking vessel (pot, pan, bowl, blender, etc.)

30 Minutes: Takes no more than 30 minutes from start to finish

Budget-Friendly: Uses inexpensive ingredients

Gluten-Free: Naturally contains no gluten

Time-Saver: Uses convenience items, such as canned, frozen, or precut vegetables

Vegan: Uses no animal products

Vegetarian: Uses no meat

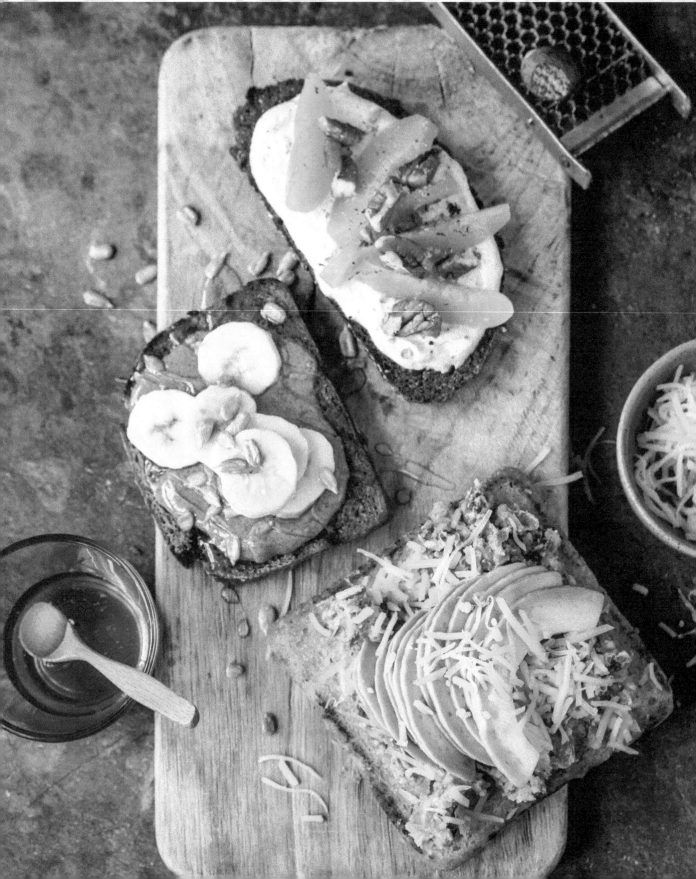

chapter four

BREAKFASTS AND SMOOTHIES

Everything Egg Scramble

30 MINUTES | BUDGET-FRIENDLY | VEGETARIAN

SERVES 3 TO 4

PREP TIME:
10 MINUTES

COOK TIME:
10 MINUTES

Per serving
Calories: 198
Total Fat: 13g
Saturated Fat: 4g
Cholesterol: 314mg
Sodium: 208mg
Carbohydrates: 8g
Fiber: 3g
Protein: 15g

This recipe could also be called a "use-it-up scramble," because you can make it with whatever veggies you have in the vegetable drawer of your refrigerator. There are no rules—just include three to four vegetables to help you hit your recommended five to six servings a day. Spinach is always a good choice; it's available year-round and is a powerhouse vegetable with generous amounts of magnesium, calcium, potassium, and fiber that help control blood pressure.

5 eggs

2 tablespoons nonfat or low-fat milk

1 teaspoon garlic powder

½ teaspoon dried basil

½ teaspoon dried oregano

¼ teaspoon freshly ground black pepper

Splash hot sauce (such as Frank's RedHot)

2 teaspoons extra-virgin olive oil

1½ cups chopped mushrooms

¼ cup finely chopped red bell pepper

¼ cup finely chopped red or green onion

1 (6-ounce) bag spinach

2 tablespoons shredded low-fat Cheddar cheese

1. In a large bowl, whisk together the eggs, milk, garlic powder, basil, oregano, black pepper, and hot sauce until fluffy.
2. Brush a medium skillet evenly with the oil and place over medium-low heat. Sauté the mushrooms, red bell pepper, and onion for about 3 minutes. Add the spinach, and toss for 2 to 3 minutes until it wilts.
3. Reduce the heat to low. Pour the egg mixture into the skillet and mix. Cook until the eggs are almost done, about 3 minutes, turning over with a rubber spatula every minute.
4. Gently mix in the Cheddar cheese. Serve immediately.

Homemade Muesli

1 POT | 30 MINUTES | VEGAN

**MAKES
16 SERVINGS**

PREP TIME:
5 MINUTES

Per serving
(½ cup)
Calories: 227
Total Fat: 14g
Saturated Fat: 1g
Cholesterol: 0mg
Sodium: 0mg
Carbohydrates: 21g
Fiber: 5g
Protein: 7g

Keep this assembly-only recipe on hand for a cereal without any added sugar or salt. It's delicious as a cold cereal with milk (and fruit, if you like), in yogurt, or as an overnight oats option. It's also a handy snack. Muesli will keep for two to three weeks in an airtight container so you have it when you need it. Be sure to buy old-fashioned oats, which are less processed than instant.

4 cups old-fashioned oats

1 cup unsalted raw pumpkin seeds

1 cup unsalted raw sunflower seeds

1 cup unsalted sliced raw or toasted almonds

1 cup unsalted raw or toasted walnuts, chopped

¼ cup low-sugar dried cranberries

1. In a large bowl, mix together the oats, pumpkin seeds, sunflower seeds, almonds, walnuts, and dried cranberries.
2. The muesli is ready to eat. Put leftovers in an airtight container and store at room temperature for 2 to 3 weeks.

Substitution tip: Try other dried fruit such as cherries, blueberries, or apricots, and other nuts you like. Also feel free to add ¼ cup chia or hemp seeds, shredded dried coconut (no sugar added), cacao nibs, or mini chocolate chips—whatever you enjoy!

Ten-Minute Toast, Three Ways

1 POT | 30 MINUTES | BUDGET-FRIENDLY | VEGETARIAN

EACH
VARIETY
MAKES
2 SLICES
OF TOAST

PREP TIME:
5 MINUTES

Toast 1
Per serving
Calories: 530
Total Fat: 26g
Saturated Fat: 3g
Cholesterol: 0mg
Sodium: 215mg
Carbohydrates: 70g
Fiber: 14g
Protein: 17g

Toast 2
Per serving
Calories: 412
Total Fat: 14g
Saturated Fat: 5g
Cholesterol: 19mg
Sodium: 293mg
Carbohydrates: 63g
Fiber: 11g
Protein: 18g

Toast 3
Per serving
Calories: 342
Total Fat: 13g
Saturated Fat: 4g
Cholesterol: 8mg
Sodium: 309mg
Carbohydrates: 58g
Fiber: 13g
Protein: 17g

These three interesting and easy toast toppers are for lazy mornings when you don't feel like cooking but you crave something a little out of the ordinary. Any one of them will get you out of your breakfast rut, and if you're not in the habit of eating breakfast, perhaps you'll want to start!

TOAST 1: NUTTY BANANA TOAST

2 tablespoons almond butter

2 slices whole-wheat or whole-grain bread, toasted

½ banana, sliced

1 teaspoon honey

1 heaping tablespoon raw unsalted sunflower seeds

Spread 1 tablespoon of almond butter on each slice of the toast. Place the banana slices on top. Drizzle with the honey and sprinkle with the sunflower seeds. Serve immediately.

TOAST 2: PEACHES AND CREAM TOAST

¼ cup part-skim ricotta cheese

¼ teaspoon ground cinnamon

¼ teaspoon ground nutmeg

2 slices whole-wheat bread, toasted

1 (15-ounce) can sliced peaches (in their own juice, no sugar added), drained

1 tablespoon unsalted pecans, finely chopped

1. In a small bowl, mix together the ricotta cheese, cinnamon, and nutmeg.
2. Spread 2 tablespoons of the ricotta mixture on each slice of toast. Top with 4 to 6 peach slices (save the rest of the peaches for another recipe or to eat as a snack). Sprinkle with the pecans, and serve.

TOAST 3: AVOCADO BEAN TOAST

1 (7-ounce) can low-sodium pinto beans, drained and rinsed, or low-sodium low-fat refried beans of your choice

⅛ teaspoon ground cumin

Splash freshly squeezed lime juice

Splash hot sauce (such as Frank's RedHot)

2 slices whole-wheat bread, toasted

¼ avocado, thinly sliced

2 tablespoons low-fat shredded Mexican cheese blend

1. In a medium bowl, mash the beans with a fork. Add the cumin, lime juice, and hot sauce, and mix well. Heat the beans in the microwave, if you'd like, for 20 seconds.

2. Spread 2 tablespoons of the bean mixture on each slice of the toast. Place the avocado slices on top. Top with the cheese, and serve.

Blueberry Oat Muffins

30 MINUTES | VEGETARIAN

**MAKES
12 MUFFINS**

PREP TIME:
10 MINUTES

COOK TIME:
20 MINUTES

Per serving
(1 muffin)
Calories: 324
Total Fat: 12g
Saturated Fat: 1g
Cholesterol: 47mg
Sodium: 74mg
Carbohydrates: 52g
Fiber: 6g
Protein: 7g

Store-bought muffins are loaded with fat, salt, and sugar, and they're calorie bombs to boot. These tender, moist muffins, on the other hand, are great for heart health and for lowering blood pressure. Store them in the freezer (in an airtight container for up to three months) and take one out whenever you need breakfast or a snack. Thaw each muffin at room temperature or microwave 45 seconds to 1 minute from frozen before eating.

1 cup uncooked
old-fashioned oats

½ cup orange juice

3 eggs

½ cup canola oil

½ cup unsweetened applesauce

3 cups whole-wheat pastry flour

1 cup sugar

4 teaspoons baking powder

½ teaspoon baking soda

2½ cups fresh blueberries

1 teaspoon ground cinnamon
(optional)

1 tablespoon sugar for all
12 muffins (optional)

1. Preheat the oven to 400°F.
2. In a small bowl, mix the oats and orange juice. Let sit for 5 minutes.
3. In a large bowl, whisk together the eggs and oil. Add the applesauce and the oat/orange juice mixture. Add the flour, sugar, baking powder, and baking soda. Stir just until combined. Gently fold in the blueberries.
4. Line each cup of a standard muffin tin with muffin papers. Fill the muffin cups three-quarters full. Sprinkle each muffin with some of the cinnamon and sugar (if using).
5. Bake in the preheated oven for 18 minutes or until the muffins start to turn light brown on top.

Ingredient tip: Using regular whole-wheat flour will change the texture of this light muffin and it will bake differently, too, so stick with whole-wheat pastry flour.

Creamy Tropical Cinnamon-Banana Smoothie

1 POT | 30 MINUTES | VEGAN

SERVES 3

PREP TIME:
10 MINUTES

Per serving
Calories: 157
Total Fat: 3g
Saturated Fat: 0g
Cholesterol: 0mg
Sodium: 12mg
Carbohydrates: 30g
Fiber: 3g
Protein: 5g

This tropical-tasting smoothie will have you dreaming of a far-off island. The tofu may be a surprising ingredient, but it gives this smoothie its amazingly creamy texture. You'll never know it's there! Pour these smoothies into separate mason jars and keep in your refrigerator (for up to 2 days) for a quick breakfast-to-go, post-workout recovery snack, or nonalcoholic piña colada substitute at happy hour. Just stir and drink!

1½ frozen bananas

1 cup canned crushed pineapple in its own juice (no sugar added)

1 cup silken tofu

½ teaspoon ground ginger

½ teaspoon vanilla extract

½ teaspoon ground cinnamon, plus extra for serving

1. In a blender, blend the bananas, pineapple, tofu, ginger, and vanilla extract until smooth. (If the bananas aren't frozen, add ice to thicken.)
2. Pour into 3 tall glasses. Serve right away, with a dash of cinnamon on top.

Substitution tip: I love the tofu in this and I think you will, too, but you can easily substitute 1 cup plain nonfat Greek yogurt if you prefer. Add 1 or 2 teaspoons of honey to balance out the tartness.

Minty Spinach Smoothie

1 POT | 30 MINUTES | BUDGET-FRIENDLY | VEGAN

SERVES 2

PREP TIME:
5 MINUTES

Per serving
Calories: 144
Total Fat: <1g
Saturated Fat: 0g
Cholesterol: 0mg
Sodium: 343mg
Carbohydrates: 31g
Fiber: 8g
Protein: 6g

The fresh minty flavor of this gorgeous green smoothie is unusual and addicting! Sipping this delightfully zingy smoothie as a snack is a great way to add veggies to your day without even knowing it. It has a surprising (and well-hidden) ingredient not found in most smoothies: green peas!

1½ cups frozen baby leaf spinach, partially thawed

1 (12.5-ounce) can pears in their own juice

8 fresh mint leaves, plus 2 sprigs for garnish

¾ cup water

⅓ cup finely chopped celery

⅓ cup frozen green peas

2 teaspoons freshly squeezed lime juice

2 teaspoons hot sauce (such as Frank's RedHot)

1. In a blender, blend the spinach, pears, mint leaves, water, celery, peas, lime juice, and hot sauce until smooth.
2. Pour into 2 tall glasses. Serve right away, garnished with a sprig of mint.

Substitution tip: If you don't like mint, try using 8 leaves of fresh basil instead.

Orange-Berry Swirl

1 POT | 30 MINUTE | BUDGET-FRIENDLY | VEGETARIAN

SERVES 2

PREP TIME:
5 MINUTES

Per serving
Calories: 200
Total Fat: 1g
Saturated Fat: <1g
Cholesterol: 3mg
Sodium: 67mg
Carbohydrates: 43g
Fiber: 4g
Protein: 6g

With this fresh-tasting purple smoothie, you can check off a couple of your daily fruit servings and increase your dairy intake; both help lower blood pressure. No elaborate ingredients here—just milk and 100 percent fruit juice, with no added sugar. To make it vegan, just substitute soy milk for the dairy milk.

2 cups frozen blueberries, no sugar added

1¼ cups nonfat milk

½ cup orange juice, no sugar added

3 tablespoons frozen orange juice concentrate, no sugar added (do not thaw)

1. In a blender, blend the blueberries, milk, orange juice, and orange juice concentrate until smooth.
2. Pour into 2 tall glasses. Serve immediately.

Ingredient tip: Blueberries contain anthocyanins, which have been found to lower blood pressure, both in the short term and long term.

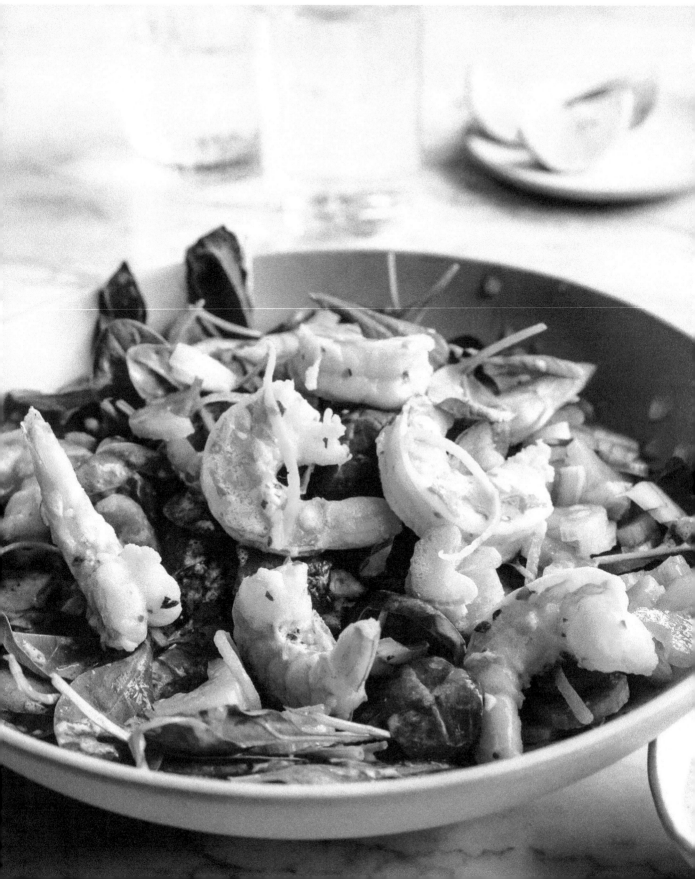

chapter five

SOUPS, SALADS, AND SIDES

◀ Citrus Shrimp and
Spinach Salad, *page 62*

Vegan Mushroom Barley Soup

1 POT | BUDGET-FRIENDLY | VEGAN

SERVES 3

PREP TIME:
20 MINUTES

COOK TIME:
45 MINUTES

Per serving
Calories: 267
Total Fat: 15g
Saturated Fat: 1g
Cholesterol: 0mg
Sodium: 187mg
Carbohydrates: 31g
Fiber: 8g
Protein: 6g

Barley, a fiber-rich whole grain, adds a pleasing chewy texture to this comforting and satisfying soup. In combination with the potassium-rich mushrooms, it creates an almost "meaty" flavor that's hard to beat. Serve with a whole-grain roll and a green salad for a perfect winter meal.

3 tablespoons canola oil

8 ounces cremini mushrooms, roughly chopped

3 large carrots, diced

2 or 3 celery stalks, diced

½ cup diced yellow onion

¼ cup pearl barley, rinsed

1 tablespoon flour

1 (14.5-ounce) can low-sodium vegetable broth

½ cup water

1 teaspoon dried dill

1 teaspoon dried marjoram

1 teaspoon dried thyme

¼ teaspoon freshly ground black pepper

1. Brush the bottom and sides of a large pot or Dutch oven with the canola oil. Heat the pot over medium-low heat.
2. Add the mushrooms, carrots, celery, onion, and barley to the pot and sauté, stirring often, until the vegetables are just about tender, 20 minutes. Add the flour to the pot and stir as it browns, 3 to 4 minutes.
3. Turn up the heat to medium. Gradually stir in the broth and water. Bring the soup to a gentle boil, stirring frequently to release all the tasty browned bits from the bottom of the pot.

4. Add the dill, marjoram, and thyme to the mixture. Reduce the heat to low, and simmer until the barley is tender and the soup begins to thicken, about 20 minutes.
5. Season with black pepper before serving. Serve hot.

Ingredient tip: Barley is an economical whole grain. You can get a whole 16-ounce bag for under a dollar on sale. This soup is not only healthy, it's also easy on the pocketbook.

Signature Spicy (or Not) Chili

1 POT | 30 MINUTES | BUDGET-FRIENDLY | TIME-SAVER

SERVES 8

PREP TIME:
10 MINUTES

COOK TIME:
25 MINUTES

Per serving
Calories: 265
Total Fat: 6g
Saturated Fat: 2g
Cholesterol: 35mg
Sodium: 115mg
Carbohydrates: 33g
Fiber: 9g
Protein: 20g

You can make this simple but delicious chili in no time with a well-stocked pantry full of these canned ingredients. The tomatoes and beans are a good source of potassium, and the lycopene in the tomatoes gives you an anti-inflammatory health benefit. Canned tomatoes have more lycopene than fresh tomatoes!

2 teaspoons canola oil

1 pound 93% lean ground beef or ground turkey

1 cup chopped yellow onion

1½ to 2 cups water

2 (15.5-ounce) cans crushed tomatoes, with their juice (no salt added)

1 (14.5-ounce) can low-sodium diced tomatoes

8 ounces tomato sauce (no salt added)

1 (6-ounce) can tomato paste (no salt added)

3 to 4 tablespoons chili powder

1 (15.5-ounce) can low-sodium black beans, drained and rinsed

1 (15.5-ounce) can low-sodium pinto beans (or kidney beans), drained and rinsed

1 (4-ounce) can green diced chiles, drained and rinsed

2 tablespoons ground cumin

1 teaspoon dried oregano

¼ teaspoon cayenne pepper

1. Evenly brush the bottom and sides of a large pot with the canola oil. Heat the pot over medium heat.
2. Add the ground meat and stir, breaking it apart with a long-handled wooden spoon as you stir. Add the chopped onion and cook, stirring frequently, until the meat is browned and cooked through, about 5 minutes.

3. Add 1½ cups of water, crushed tomatoes, diced tomatoes, tomato sauce, tomato paste, and chili powder to the pot and bring to a boil. Stir in the black beans, pinto beans, diced chiles, cumin, oregano, and cayenne pepper. Add the remaining ½ cup of water, if needed. Reduce the heat to medium-low, and simmer for about 20 minutes, stirring occasionally. Serve hot.

Serving tip: Serve with nonfat plain Greek yogurt, chopped scallions, shredded low-fat cheese, and/or chopped avocado.

Fireside Beef Stew

1 POT | BUDGET-FRIENDLY

SERVES 4 TO 6

PREP TIME:
20 MINUTES

COOK TIME:
1 HOUR,
10 MINUTES

Per 4 servings
Calories: 385
Total Fat: 10g
Saturated Fat: 2g
Cholesterol: 75mg
Sodium: 207mg
Carbohydrates: 38g
Fiber: 9g
Protein: 33g

This belly-warming, braise-in-the-oven beef stew hits the spot after a winter activity or when you'd rather watch a movie than fuss in the kitchen. The tender chunks of beef with the deep flavors from the wine are a crowd-pleaser, especially when served with some crusty whole-grain bread and a side salad. This stew freezes and reheats well, so double the batch and keep another meal in the freezer.

¼ cup all-purpose flour

½ teaspoon dried thyme

½ teaspoon dried oregano

1 pound beef stew meat

2 teaspoons canola oil, plus 1 teaspoon

3 garlic cloves, chopped

2 (14.5-ounce) cans low-sodium whole tomatoes, in their juice

½ (6-ounce) can tomato paste, no salt added

½ cup green peas

1½ cups water, plus more if needed

½ cup good-quality red wine (cabernet or merlot)

3 large carrots, cut into coins

1 (8-ounce) package small whole mushrooms, such as cremini

3 large celery stalks, chopped

½ (14.4-ounce) bag frozen white pearl onions

1 to 2 dried bay leaves

1. Preheat the oven to 375°F.
2. In a sealable plastic bag, combine the flour, thyme, and oregano. Add the stew meat and shake to coat.
3. Evenly brush the bottom and sides of a large Dutch oven with 2 teaspoons of canola oil.
4. Add the stew meat to the pot, and brown the meat over medium heat, 3 to 4 minutes, stirring occasionally. Add the chopped garlic to the stew meat and cook for 1 minute.

5. Add the tomatoes, tomato paste, and peas, and stir well, adding 1 tablespoon of water, and using a wooden spoon, scrape the bottom of the pan to stir up all the flavorful browned bits.

6. Add the remaining water, wine, carrots, mushrooms, celery, pearl onions, and bay leaves to the mixture. Stir well.

7. Bake in the preheated oven for 1 hour. Remove and discard the bay leaves before serving.

Ingredient tip: Use a lean cut of beef such as round or sirloin when it's on sale, and cut it into 1-inch to 1½-inch chunks. The long, slow cooking process of this recipe makes even tougher cuts of meat tender and juicy.

Moroccan Kale and Bulgur Salad

BUDGET-FRIENDLY | VEGAN

SERVES 4

PREP TIME:
20 MINUTES

COOK TIME:
15 MINUTES

Per serving
Calories: 371
Total Fat: 21g
Saturated Fat: 3g
Cholesterol: 0mg
Sodium: 33mg
Carbohydrates: 44g
Fiber: 9g
Protein: 8g

This flavorful greens-and-grains salad will delight you with its delicious, nutty-tasting whole grain: bulgur. It's a type of fast-cooking cracked wheat that's high in fiber and equal in protein to quinoa. If you can't find bulgur, quinoa is a great substitute.

FOR THE SALAD

2 cups water

1 cup bulgur

2 teaspoons extra-virgin olive oil

2 teaspoons freshly squeezed lemon juice

1 small bunch lacinato kale, stemmed and cut into ribbons

½ cup finely chopped scallions

¼ cup fresh basil, cut into ribbons

¼ cup grated carrots (store-bought is fine)

¼ cup golden raisins

3 to 4 tablespoons toasted sliced almonds

FOR THE DRESSING

¼ cup extra-virgin olive oil

2 or 3 garlic cloves, finely chopped

1 teaspoon fresh lemon zest

1 tablespoon freshly squeezed lemon juice

1 teaspoon honey

½ teaspoon ground cumin

½ teaspoon ground coriander

To make the salad

1. In a medium pot over medium-high heat, combine the water and the bulgur. Bring to a boil, cover, then reduce the heat and simmer until tender, about 12 minutes. Drain off any excess liquid and fluff the bulgur with a fork. Let cool.
2. In a large bowl, massage the olive oil and lemon juice into the kale ribbons for 1 to 2 minutes.
3. Add the cooled bulgur to the kale.
4. Add the scallions, basil, carrots, raisins, and almonds, and stir together gently.

To make the dressing

1. In a small bowl, whisk together the olive oil, garlic, and lemon zest.

2. Add the lemon juice, honey, cumin, and coriander, and whisk until well combined.

3. Add 3 tablespoons of dressing to the salad and toss well before serving. (Add more dressing if you like.) Store leftover dressing in an airtight jar in the refrigerator for up to 2 weeks.

Preparation tip: Here's a quick way to prepare the kale: Grip the stalk and run your fingers quickly downward to remove the leaves. Discard the stems. Stack the leaves and slice them into 1-inch ribbons. Then wash and dry the kale.

Mediterranean Quinoa Salad

30 MINUTES | GLUTEN-FREE | VEGAN

SERVES 4

PREP TIME:
10 MINUTES

COOK TIME:
15 MINUTES

Per serving
Calories: 439
Total Fat: 15g
Saturated Fat: 2g
Cholesterol: 0mg
Sodium: 12mg
Carbohydrates: 64g
Fiber: 10g
Protein: 14g

This salad is quick, colorful, and high in protein because of the chick-peas and the quinoa. Quinoa is an ancient whole grain chock-full of blood pressure–lowering magnesium and fiber. Serve this as a side salad, or in a pita pocket or a lettuce cup as an appetizer.

1 cup tricolor quinoa, rinsed and drained

1½ cups water

1 (15.5-ounce) can low-sodium chickpeas, drained and rinsed

1 (14-ounce) can quartered artichokes, drained and rinsed

1 cup cherry tomatoes, halved

1 red bell pepper, chopped

1 cup peeled, chopped cucumber

½ cup finely chopped red onion

3 tablespoons extra-virgin olive oil

3 tablespoons freshly squeezed lemon juice

1 teaspoon garlic powder

½ teaspoon dried basil

1 teaspoon fresh lemon zest

Freshly ground black pepper

2 tablespoons fresh parsley, for garnish

1. In a medium pot over medium-low heat, bring the quinoa and water to a boil. Reduce the heat to low and cook until all the liquid is absorbed, about 15 minutes. Let sit, covered, for 5 minutes, then remove the lid and let cool.
2. In a large bowl, combine the chickpeas, artichokes, cherry toma-toes, red bell pepper, cucumber, and red onion. Add the cooled quinoa and stir.
3. In a separate small bowl, whisk together the olive oil, lemon juice, garlic powder, basil, and lemon zest. Season with black pepper.
4. Before serving, pour the dressing over the quinoa salad, toss to combine, and sprinkle with the parsley.

Spring Greens with Apricots, Goat Cheese, and Sizzled Shallots

30 MINUTES | GLUTEN-FREE | VEGETARIAN

SERVES 4

PREP TIME:
5 MINUTES

COOK TIME:
15 MINUTES

Per serving
Calories: 161
Total Fat: 7g
Saturated Fat: 1g
Cholesterol: 3mg
Sodium: 37mg
Carbohydrates: 21g
Fiber: 2g
Protein: 4g

This unique salad, with its sharp, tart, sweet flavors and crispy shallots, just might become your go-to dish for weeknights and for entertaining. Skip store-bought dressings loaded with salt and unhealthy fats, and make your own Everyday Herb Vinaigrette (page 163) or use a simple mix of olive oil and red-wine vinegar.

2 teaspoons canola oil, for the pan

4 large shallots, cut into thin rings and separated

½ bag prewashed spring greens mix

4 to 6 dried apricots, finely chopped

2 tablespoons crumbled goat cheese

2 to 3 tablespoons Everyday Herb Vinaigrette (page 163),

2 tablespoons unsalted, shelled sunflower seeds

1. Evenly brush a small skillet with the canola oil and heat the pan over medium heat. Add the shallots and sauté, stirring often, until they're brown and crispy, about 15 minutes. Transfer to a paper towel-lined plate.
2. In a large salad bowl, combine the spring greens, apricots, and goat cheese. Add the shallots. Add the herb vinaigrette and toss well. Sprinkle the sunflower seeds on top for a nutty finish.

Citrus Shrimp and Spinach Salad

GLUTEN-FREE

SERVES 4

PREP TIME:
35 MINUTES
(PLUS 1 TO
3 HOURS TO
MARINATE)

COOK TIME:
10 MINUTES

Per serving
Calories: 294
Total Fat: 20g
Saturated Fat: 3g
Cholesterol: 166mg
Sodium: 239mg
Carbohydrates: 10g
Fiber: 1g
Protein: 21g

This light, fresh dish is the perfect choice for a summertime lunch or dinner—or anytime you're craving a succulent seafood salad. The vibrant citrus marinade and vinaigrette is just what shrimp needs to bring out its flavor. And the spinach has loads of potassium, so you'll be doing your blood pressure a favor.

FOR THE SHRIMP

1 pound frozen raw shrimp, thawed

¼ cup extra-virgin olive oil, plus 2 teaspoons

¼ cup freshly squeezed lemon juice

¼ cup orange juice

2 tablespoons freshly squeezed lime juice

2 garlic cloves, finely chopped

2 teaspoons packed brown sugar

1 teaspoon fresh lemon zest

¾ teaspoon dried basil

¼ teaspoon red pepper flakes

FOR THE SALAD

¼ cup nonfat plain Greek yogurt

1 tablespoon extra-virgin olive oil

1 teaspoon sweet chili sauce

½ (6-ounce) bag fresh baby spinach

¼ red onion, sliced

¼ cup sliced celery

To make the shrimp

1. Drain the thawed shrimp. If necessary (check the package), remove the shells and tails, and devein. Rinse the shrimp and drain again. Pat dry with a paper towel.
2. In a small bowl, combine ¼ cup of olive oil with the lemon juice, orange juice, and lime juice. Add the garlic, brown sugar, lemon zest, dried basil, and red pepper flakes, and whisk until well blended.
3. Combine the raw shrimp and the marinade in a medium bowl and stir well. Marinate the shrimp for 1 to 3 hours in the refrigerator.

4. Transfer the shrimp to a plate, reserving the marinade in a small saucepan.
5. Brush the bottom of a medium sauté pan with the remaining 2 teaspoons of olive oil. Heat the pan over medium-low heat. Do not let the oil burn.
6. Add the shrimp and cook without stirring until white and pink, 1 to 2 minutes. (Watch carefully because shrimp cooks very quickly.) Flip and cook another 1 to 2 minutes. Transfer immediately to a paper towel–lined plate to cool.

To make the salad
1. Over medium-high heat, bring the reserved marinade to a boil. Boil vigorously, stirring occasionally, until the marinade is reduced to ½ cup, about 5 minutes. (This will kill any bacteria from the raw shrimp.) Remove from the heat and let cool.
2. Whisk the yogurt, olive oil, and sweet chili sauce into the marinade. Chill for at least 15 minutes. Stir before using.
3. Put the spinach in a large salad bowl with the shrimp. Add the onion, celery, and 3 tablespoons of the marinade dressing, and toss until well combined. Add more dressing, if desired, before serving.

Preparation tip: To save time, thaw and prep the shrimp and make the dressing the day before, so the salad is ready to assemble.

Garlic Roasted Red Potatoes

30 MINUTES | BUDGET-FRIENDLY | GLUTEN-FREE | VEGAN

SERVES 4

PREP TIME:
5 MINUTES

COOK TIME:
25 MINUTES

Per serving
Calories: 148
Total Fat: 7g
Saturated Fat: 1g
Cholesterol: 0mg
Sodium: 1mg
Carbohydrates: 21g
Fiber: 2g
Protein: 2g

This simple side dish is great to serve with your favorite protein and is a snap to prepare! These simple ingredients take ordinary potatoes to a flavor level you won't want to miss—no salt needed! Potatoes are inexpensive and a good source of potassium, which has been shown to help control blood pressure.

1 pound small red new potatoes, cut into quarters

2 tablespoons extra-virgin olive oil

2 garlic cloves, minced

2 teaspoons dried rosemary or 2 tablespoons fresh rosemary

¼ teaspoon freshly ground black pepper

1. Preheat the oven to 400°F.
2. In a large mixing bowl, place the potatoes, olive oil, garlic, rosemary, and pepper, and toss to combine.
3. On a large baking sheet, spread the potato mixture evenly, leaving space between the potato quarters so they have room to brown. Roast for 25 minutes, stirring once about halfway through the baking time. Serve hot.

Ingredient tip: Feel free to use any variety of potato, except Yukon Gold, which has a higher moisture content and doesn't brown as quickly.

Charred Stovetop Broccoli

1 POT | 30 MINUTES | BUDGET-FRIENDLY | GLUTEN-FREE | VEGAN

SERVES 4

PREP TIME:
5 MINUTES

COOK TIME:
10 MINUTES

Per serving
Calories: 43
Total Fat: 3g
Saturated Fat: <1g
Cholesterol: 0mg
Sodium: 21mg
Carbohydrates: 4g
Fiber: 2g
Protein: 2g

My husband is the one who discovered the unique broccoli preparation for this recipe. The charred flavor is a nice change from steamed or roasted broccoli. Broccoli is a good source of potassium, along with a host of other healthy nutrients, so enjoy it regularly. This recipe uses the entire crown of broccoli with the stalks included, so there's no waste.

2 medium crowns fresh broccoli, cut into spears (including the stalks)

¾ cup water

2 teaspoons extra-virgin olive oil

1 to 2 teaspoons freshly squeezed lemon juice

½ teaspoon garlic powder

Freshly ground black pepper

1. In a large sauté pan, place the broccoli and water. Cover and bring to a boil over medium heat, stirring occasionally, until the water has completely evaporated, 5 to 7 minutes. Once the water is evaporated, stir to brown all sides of the broccoli.
2. Remove from the heat. Drizzle the broccoli with the olive oil and lemon juice, sprinkle with the garlic powder, and toss to coat well. Season with pepper before serving.

Roasted Root Vegetable Medley

1 POT | BUDGET-FRIENDLY | VEGAN

SERVES 4

PREP TIME:
15 MINUTES

COOK TIME:
25 MINUTES

Per serving
Calories: 169
Total Fat: 10g
Saturated Fat: 1g
Cholesterol: 0mg
Sodium: 30mg
Carbohydrates: 19g
Fiber: 4g
Protein: 2g

All the veggies in this recipe, except for the onion, are what we call starchy vegetables, but they're nutrition powerhouses. Roasting them brings out a complex sweetness that may surprise you. Serve this dish as a vegetable side for weeknight dinners or holidays, or as healthy "vegetable fries" alongside a sandwich or salad.

2 carrots, peeled and cut into 3-by-1-inch sticks

1 medium sweet potato, peeled and cut into 3-by-1-inch sticks

1 large parsnip, peeled and cut into 3-by-1-inch sticks

½ large red onion, sliced

2 tablespoons plus 2 teaspoons avocado oil (or other high-heat oil such as peanut oil)

Splash white balsamic vinegar

1. Preheat the oven to 425°F.
2. On a large baking pan, toss the carrots, sweet potato, parsnip, and onion together with the avocado oil. Spread out evenly.
3. Roast for 25 minutes, using tongs to stir twice during the roasting.
4. Splash with vinegar before serving.

Sensational Sautéed Greens

1 POT | 30 MINUTES | BUDGET-FRIENDLY | TIME-SAVER | VEGAN

SERVES 4

PREP TIME:
10 MINUTES

COOK TIME:
10 MINUTES

Per serving
Calories: 49
Total Fat: 3g
Saturated Fat: <1g
Cholesterol: 0mg
Sodium: 1mg
Carbohydrates: 3g
Fiber: 2g
Protein: 2g

Kale came into vogue several years ago, and there's been no stopping it. Why? Because it delivers so much nutrition—B vitamins, potassium, and vitamin K—and so much flavor! The beautiful bright color and tender texture (yes, curly kale can be tender) of the kale in this recipe will add interest to your plates.

2 teaspoons extra-virgin olive oil

¼ cup sliced sweet onion

2 or 3 garlic cloves, chopped

1 (8-ounce) bag prewashed, precut curly kale

½ cup water

1 to 2 tablespoons white balsamic vinegar

Freshly ground black pepper

1. Brush the bottom of a sauté pan evenly with the olive oil. Heat over medium heat. Add the onion and sauté until translucent, 2 to 3 minutes. Add the garlic, stir, and cook for another 2 minutes.
2. Add the kale and water. Cook for 5 minutes, covered, until the kale turns bright green.
3. Splash the kale with the vinegar and season with pepper before serving.

Mandarin Orange, Arugula, and Almond Salad

30 MINUTES | BUDGET-FRIENDLY | TIME-SAVER | VEGAN

SERVES 4

PREP TIME:
10 MINUTES

Per serving
Calories: 154
Total Fat: 14g
Saturated Fat: 2g
Cholesterol: 0mg
Sodium: 6mg
Carbohydrates: 9g
Fiber: 2g
Protein: 2g

This salad comes together in minutes because it's made from convenience items. Arugula is one of my favorite high-potassium leafy greens and is among the most important vegetables to include in your daily diet to support a healthy blood pressure.

1 (10-ounce) can mandarin oranges in their own juice (no syrup or added sugar)

3 tablespoons extra-virgin olive oil

1 tablespoon white balsamic vinegar

½ (7-ounce) bag prewashed arugula

¼ cup unsalted toasted sliced or slivered almonds

Freshly ground black pepper

1. Drain the mandarin oranges, reserving 4½ tablespoons of the juice.
2. In a small bowl, whisk together the olive oil, vinegar, and the reserved juice to make the dressing.
3. In a large salad bowl, toss together the arugula, drained oranges, and almonds. Add 2 to 3 tablespoons of the dressing (or more if you prefer) and toss to coat.

White Bean and Cabbage Soup

1 POT | BUDGET-FRIENDLY | TIME-SAVER

SERVES 4

PREP TIME:
15 MINUTES

COOK TIME:
25 MINUTES

Per serving
Calories: 292
Total Fat: 3g
Saturated Fat: <1g
Cholesterol: 0mg
Sodium: 105mg
Carbohydrates: 53g
Fiber: 20g
Protein: 16g

This low-carb soup is a cinch to prepare because it uses primarily precut or canned ingredients from your pantry. It's a good soup to take for a healthy work lunch or to eat on a weight-loss plan. It also has the added benefit of the fiber from the beans to lower your blood pressure and keep you satisfied for hours.

2 teaspoons canola oil

2 garlic cloves, finely chopped

2 celery stalks, finely chopped

½ cup finely chopped sweet onion

3 carrots, cut into coins

1 (16-ounce) bag preshredded cabbage

1 (14.5-ounce) can low-sodium chicken broth

1½ cups water

2 (15.5-ounce) cans low-sodium white navy beans, rinsed and drained

2 dried bay leaves

2 tablespoons herbes de Provence

1. Evenly brush the bottom and sides of a large pot with the canola oil. Heat the pot over medium heat. Add the garlic, celery, and onion, and sauté until soft, 3 to 4 minutes. Add the carrots and cabbage, stirring to combine.
2. Pour in the broth and water. Mix in the beans, bay leaves, and the herbes de Provence. Bring to a low boil, reduce the heat to low, and gently simmer, stirring occasionally, for 15 to 20 minutes. Remove and discard the bay leaves before serving.

Ingredient tip: You can make this recipe vegan by using low-sodium vegetable broth instead of the chicken broth.

Butternut Squash and Cannellini Bean Soup

BUDGET-FRIENDLY | TIME-SAVER | VEGETARIAN

SERVES 4

PREP TIME:
15 MINUTES

COOK TIME:
30 MINUTES

Per serving
Calories: 200
Total Fat: 3g
Saturated Fat: <1g
Cholesterol: <1mg
Sodium: 45mg
Carbohydrates: 38g
Fiber: 12g
Protein: 8g

This creamy and rich-tasting soup makes a great lunch or light dinner along with a salad and a whole-wheat roll. Using high-potassium, high-fiber beans is an easy way to add plant protein to your diet. The amazingly silky mouthfeel of this soup comes from the beans' soluble fiber when it's blended with the other ingredients.

1 small butternut squash

2 teaspoons extra-virgin olive oil

1 medium yellow onion, diced

1 (15.5-ounce) can low-sodium cannellini beans, drained and rinsed

1 cup low-sodium vegetable broth

⅔ cup water

¼ cup apple juice

2 teaspoons apple-cider vinegar, plus 1 teaspoon

1½ teaspoons ground ginger

2 tablespoons nonfat plain Greek yogurt, for garnish

2 tablespoons chopped fresh chives, for garnish

1. Cut the butternut squash into two halves lengthwise. Place the halves cut-side down in a glass dish and cook for 15 minutes in the microwave until very soft. Remove and cool.
2. Evenly brush a large skillet with the olive oil. Add the onion and sauté over medium heat until translucent, 3 to 4 minutes. Stir in the beans and cook for another 3 to 4 minutes.
3. Add 2 cups of the cooked squash, the broth, water, apple juice, 2 teaspoons of vinegar, and the ginger, and stir until well combined. Cook for 3 to 4 minutes to combine the flavors. Stir again.

4. Using a blender, purée the soup in batches until smooth.
5. Stir in the remaining 1 teaspoon of vinegar.
6. Top each serving with a dollop of Greek yogurt and a sprinkling of chives.

Ingredient tip: Butternut squash can keep for a few months, so you can buy it when it's in season and make this soup later. You can also buy peeled, precut butternut squash to speed up prep and cooking time. The precut cubes will only take 5 to 10 minutes in the microwave to become fork-tender.

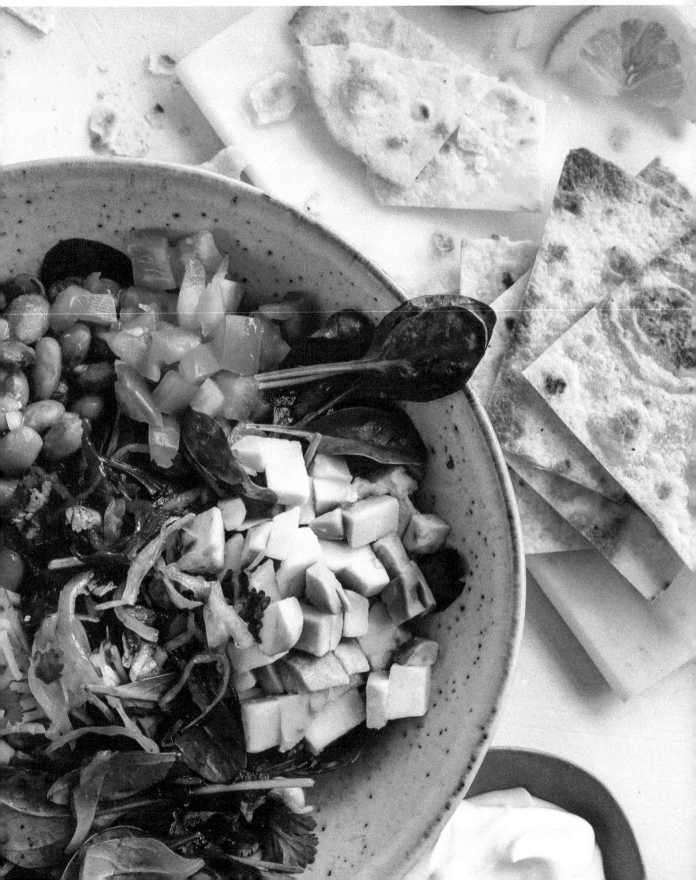

chapter six

MEATLESS MAINS

Lentils Bolognese with Red Wine

GLUTEN-FREE | VEGAN

SERVES 4

PREP TIME:
20 MINUTES

COOK TIME:
35 MINUTES

Per serving
Calories: 211
Total Fat: 3g
Saturated Fat: <1g
Cholesterol: 0mg
Sodium: 60mg
Carbohydrates: 30g
Fiber: 10g
Protein: 9g

Served over pappardelle noodles or brown rice, this recipe is perfect for fall, winter, or anytime you have red wine on hand. Lentils are a hearty, easy-to-cook legume, and they don't require any soaking time like many other dried beans do. This dish tastes like you've gone to a lot of trouble in the kitchen, but it's really very simple to prepare. Keep that a secret!

½ cup dried lentils

¾ cup plus 2 tablespoons water, plus ½ cup

1 cup red wine, divided

2 teaspoons extra-virgin olive oil

½ cup finely chopped red onion

½ red bell pepper, finely chopped

½ cup grated carrot

2 large garlic cloves, finely chopped

⅛ teaspoon red pepper flakes (optional)

1 (15.5-ounce) crushed tomatoes, with their juice (no salt added)

1 tablespoon drained, finely chopped sun-dried tomatoes

½ tablespoon dried oregano

½ teaspoon dried thyme

1 tablespoon tomato paste (no salt added)

¼ teaspoon freshly ground black pepper

1. Measure out the lentils and sort through them to remove any debris or pebbles. Wash them in a sieve and drain. In a medium saucepan, over medium heat, heat the lentils, ¾ cup plus 2 tablespoons of water, and ½ cup of wine. Cook the lentils until all the liquid is absorbed, about 20 minutes.

2. In a medium sauté pan over medium heat, brush the oil evenly onto the bottom and sides of the pan. Add the onion, red bell pepper, and carrot, and sauté for 3 to 4 minutes. Stir in the garlic and red pepper flakes (if using), and cook for about 1 minute.

3. Add to the pan the remaining ½ cup of water, the remaining ½ cup of wine, crushed tomatoes, sun-dried tomatoes, oregano, thyme, and tomato paste. Season with the black pepper, and stir well to combine. Simmer the mixture for 10 minutes, adding a little more water if needed. Stir in the cooked lentils, reduce the heat to low, and heat until the mixture is warm.

Ingredient tip: I don't recommend using canned lentils for this recipe, because they'll become too mushy.

Sesame, Tofu, and Bok Choy Stir-Fry

BUDGET-FRIENDLY | GLUTEN-FREE | VEGAN

SERVES 4

PREP TIME:
10 TO
15 MINUTES
(PLUS 6 TO
8 HOURS TO
MARINATE)

COOK TIME:
10 MINUTES

Per serving
Calories: 259
Total Fat: 16g
Saturated Fat: 2g
Cholesterol: 0mg
Sodium: 84mg
Carbohydrates: 20g
Fiber: 3g
Protein: 14g

Tofu is made of pressed soybeans, and research has shown it delivers many health benefits. It helps to lower blood pressure and LDL ("bad") cholesterol levels, provides iron and high-quality plant protein, and even protects against some cancers, cardiovascular disease, and osteoporosis. Because it's a complete protein, tofu can be used instead of meat in a variety of dishes. A stir-fry is a great way to try it out!

FOR THE TOFU

1 (12- to 14-ounce) block extra-firm tofu

2 tablespoons frozen orange juice concentrate (do not add water)

1 tablespoon avocado oil

1 tablespoon grated, peeled fresh ginger

2 teaspoons rice vinegar

1½ teaspoons toasted sesame oil

1 teaspoon finely chopped garlic

1 teaspoon sesame seeds

FOR THE STIR-FRY

1 heaping tablespoon frozen orange juice concentrate (do not add water)

1 teaspoon rice vinegar, plus 1 tablespoon

1 teaspoon toasted sesame oil

1 teaspoon sriracha hot sauce, plus extra for serving

2 teaspoons avocado oil (or peanut oil)

1 medium zucchini, cut in half lengthwise, then cut into half-moons

1 cup sliced red onion

½ orange, red, or yellow bell pepper, cut into strips

Leaves of 4 or 5 small bok choy (or 1 large head bok choy)

½ (8-ounce) package mushrooms (any kind), roughly chopped

2 tablespoons sesame seeds

To make the tofu

1. Place the tofu between paper towels and set a heavy pot on top for about 5 minutes to remove the excess water. Cut the pressed tofu into 1-inch cubes.
2. In a small bowl, put the frozen orange juice concentrate, avocado oil, ginger, vinegar, sesame oil, garlic, and sesame seeds. Whisk together until well combined. Pour into a glass casserole dish and add the tofu cubes, gently stirring to coat all the cubes with the marinade. Cover and refrigerate overnight or as long as possible.

To make the stir-fry

1. In a small bowl, combine the orange juice concentrate, 1 teaspoon of vinegar, sesame oil, and sriracha to make the stir-fry sauce. Set aside.
2. Over medium-high heat, brush the avocado oil evenly onto the bottom and sides of a wok or large skillet. Add the zucchini, onion, and bell pepper to the pan, and sprinkle with the remaining 1 tablespoon of vinegar. Stir-fry, tossing the mixture together gently for 3 minutes. Then add the bok choy and mushrooms, and stir-fry for another 3 to 4 minutes.
3. Push the mixture to the side of the pan and add the drained tofu cubes. Cook the tofu over medium-low heat for about 2 minutes. Then add the stir-fry sauce and gently toss to combine. Do not overcook—the vegetables should be crisp-tender.
4. Serve with extra sriracha on the side.

Two-Bean Cocoa Chili

**1 POT | 30 MINUTES | BUDGET-FRIENDLY | GLUTEN-FREE
TIME-SAVER | VEGETARIAN**

SERVES 4

PREP TIME:
15 MINUTES

COOK TIME:
15 MINUTES

Per serving
Calories: 322
Total Fat: 4g
Saturated Fat: <1g
Cholesterol: 1mg
Sodium: 169mg
Carbohydrates: 56g
Fiber: 14g
Protein: 18g

The creative and complex flavor of this chili comes partly from a surprise ingredient: cocoa powder! Cocoa powder contains antioxidants that can lower inflammation in the body. This is a good dish if you want a robust chili that fills you up . . . and warms you up! Double the recipe if you want to save some for another day; it freezes well.

2 teaspoons canola oil

1 small yellow onion, chopped

2 tablespoons chili powder

1½ tablespoons unsweetened cocoa powder

1 tablespoon ground cumin

1 teaspoon garlic powder

1 (15.5-ounce) can low-sodium light red kidney beans, rinsed and drained

1 (15.5-ounce) can low-sodium black beans, rinsed and drained

1 (14.5-ounce) can crushed tomatoes, with their juice (no salt added)

1 (14.5-ounce) can diced tomatoes, with their juice (no salt added)

1 (4-ounce) can chopped green chiles, drained but not rinsed

1½ cups water

1 teaspoon dried basil

1 teaspoon dried oregano

4 ounces nonfat plain Greek yogurt (or low-fat sour cream), for garnish

4 scallions, chopped, for garnish

1. Brush the bottom and sides of a large pot or Dutch oven with the canola oil. Heat over low heat. Add the onion and sauté until soft. Add the chili powder, cocoa powder, cumin, and garlic powder, and stir with the onions until fragrant, about 1 minute.

2. Add the kidney beans, black beans, crushed tomatoes, diced tomatoes, and the green chiles. Add the water, basil, and oregano, and stir well. Simmer over medium heat for 10 minutes. Add more water, if needed, to make the consistency you like.

3. Serve with a dollop of nonfat plain Greek yogurt and the chopped scallions on top.

Ingredient tip: Check the labels on canned green chiles, because the sodium content can vary a lot among brands. I've found Rio Luna green chiles to be among the lowest in sodium (45 milligrams per 2 tablespoons).

Braised White Beans with Spinach

1 POT | 30 MINUTES | BUDGET-FRIENDLY | TIME-SAVER | VEGAN

SERVES 4

PREP TIME:
10 MINUTES

COOK TIME:
15 MINUTES

Per serving
Calories: 323
Total Fat: 9g
Saturated Fat: 1g
Cholesterol: 0mg
Sodium: 69mg
Carbohydrates: 48g
Fiber: 17g
Protein: 15g

The flavors that come together in this dish are extraordinary, especially when you consider that it's made with so few ingredients! This is a fiber-rich weeknight meal loaded with nutrition that you can feel good about serving over brown rice or whole-wheat pasta or couscous. It reheats beautifully and is even better the next day!

2 (15.5-ounce) cans low-sodium great northern beans (or cannellini beans), drained and rinsed

2 tablespoons extra-virgin olive oil, plus 1 teaspoon

⅔ cup finely chopped shallots

2 teaspoons dried thyme

5 large garlic cloves, chopped

1½ cups low-sodium vegetable broth

1 cup water

1 (7-ounce) bag fresh spinach

2 teaspoons white-wine vinegar

¼ teaspoon freshly ground black pepper

1. Mash one can of beans and set aside.
2. Over medium heat, evenly brush the bottom and sides of a large skillet with 2 tablespoons of olive oil. Add the chopped shallots and thyme, and sauté, stirring frequently, about 2 minutes, or until the shallots are soft—don't let them brown. Add the garlic and stir for 1 minute.
3. Add the mashed beans, whole beans, broth, and water. Cook over medium heat for 3 to 5 minutes, stirring well. Gently stir in the fresh spinach with tongs. The liquids will become a thickened and creamy sauce. Cook another 5 to 7 minutes, until the spinach wilts.
4. Before serving, stir in the vinegar and black pepper. Then drizzle the remaining 1 teaspoon of olive oil over the entire dish.

Spicy Chickpeas over Rice

1 POT | 30 MINUTES | GLUTEN-FREE | VEGAN

Chickpeas, which are high in fiber, are featured in this recipe because they're a wonderful foil for the tomatoes and aromatic spices that make this dish memorable. A spicy one-skillet wonder, it will satisfy your cravings for Indian cuisine at home. This recipe has a kick, so feel free to use less spice to suit your tolerance.

SERVES 4

PREP TIME:
10 MINUTES

COOK TIME:
20 MINUTES

Per serving
Calories: 524
Total Fat: 13g
Saturated Fat: 2g
Cholesterol: 0mg
Sodium: 44mg
Carbohydrates: 85g
Fiber: 17g
Protein: 19g

2 (15-ounce) cans low-sodium chickpeas

2 tablespoons extra-virgin olive oil

1½ cups chopped white onion

2 (14.5-ounce) cans diced tomatoes (no salt added)

1 teaspoon ground coriander

1 teaspoon ground cumin

½ teaspoon ground ginger

½ teaspoon paprika

¼ teaspoon cayenne pepper

1 tablespoon freshly squeezed lemon juice

3 cups cooked brown rice

1. Strain the chickpeas and reserve the juice (called aquafaba).
2. Evenly brush the bottom and sides of a skillet with the olive oil. Add the onion and sauté over medium heat until it's translucent (not brown). Add ½ cup of the reserved aquafaba, the tomatoes, coriander, cumin, ginger, paprika, and cayenne. Reduce the heat and simmer for 5 to 10 minutes.
3. Add the chickpeas and stir, simmering for 5 minutes more. (Add more of the reserved aquafaba if you need more liquid.)
4. Stir in the lemon juice, and then serve immediately over the brown rice.

Umami Mushroom and Tofu Quesadillas

30 MINUTES | GLUTEN-FREE | VEGETARIAN

MAKES 4 QUESADILLAS

PREP TIME:
15 MINUTES

COOK TIME:
15 MINUTES

Per serving
(1 quesadilla)
Calories: 478
Total Fat: 18g
Saturated Fat: 6g
Cholesterol: 21mg
Sodium: 620mg
Carbohydrates: 55g
Fiber: 7g
Protein: 29g

These quesadillas are a fantastic way to use tofu and get deep, complex flavors by adding mushrooms—an "umami," or savory, food. You can also use the quesadilla filling to stir into scrambled eggs, spread on an English muffin, or put atop slices of baguette for an appetizer. Feel free to double this recipe—it'll keep for a week in the refrigerator.

FOR THE FILLING

1 (14-ounce) block extra-firm tofu

2 teaspoons extra-virgin olive oil

1 (12-ounce) package cremini mushrooms, chopped

¾ cup chopped sweet onion

4 teaspoons red-wine vinegar

¾ cup chopped fresh basil

FOR THE QUESADILLAS

⅔ cup Greek yogurt cream cheese (or low-fat or nonfat cream cheese)

⅓ cup crumbled goat cheese (or part-skim shredded mozzarella)

2 tablespoons drained, finely chopped sun-dried tomatoes

8 (5- to 6-inch) whole-wheat tortillas

Cooking spray

To make the filling

1. Place the tofu between paper towels and set a heavy pot on top for about 5 minutes to remove the excess water. Dice the pressed tofu into small cubes.
2. Over medium heat, evenly brush the olive oil on the bottom and sides of a large sauté pan. Add the mushrooms and onion, and sauté for about 3 minutes, until the onion is translucent and the mushrooms have shrunk. Add the vinegar and the tofu. Stir gently and cook for another 3 to 4 minutes.
3. Remove from the heat and stir in the basil.

To make the quesadillas

1. Mash together the softened cream cheese, goat cheese, and sun-dried tomatoes until the mixture is smooth and spreadable. Be sure to distribute the tomatoes throughout the spread.

2. Spread 1 tablespoon of the cheese mixture on a tortilla, followed by ½ cup of the tofu mixture. Place another tortilla on top. Repeat until you have 4 quesadillas.

3. Spray a small sauté pan with cooking spray and heat on low-medium heat. Don't let it smoke or burn. Put 1 quesadilla in the pan and press it down, heating it for about 3 minutes. Then flip it over and press it down for another 3 minutes, until the tortilla begins to brown and the cheese spread begins to melt. Repeat for the other 3 quesadillas. Serve immediately.

Tangy Tofu over Noodles

BUDGET-FRIENDLY | VEGETARIAN

SERVES 4

PREP TIME:
10 MINUTES,
PLUS
30 MINUTES
TO MARINATE

COOK TIME:
25 MINUTES

Per serving
Calories: 517
Total Fat: 22g
Saturated Fat: 3g
Cholesterol: 0mg
Sodium: 45mg
Carbohydrates: 60g
Fiber: 10g
Protein: 21g

This speedy and simple tangy tofu is a riff on the popular Japanese dish of yakisoba noodles. The tofu marinade is also used as a sauce for the broccoli slaw. Adding another vegetable to this dish (such as cauliflower or broccoli) can help you hit your target vegetable intake for the day to help lower blood pressure.

1 (14-ounce) block extra-firm tofu

¼ cup extra-virgin olive oil

3 tablespoons freshly squeezed lime juice

4 garlic cloves, finely chopped

4 teaspoons honey

2 teaspoons ground cumin

1 teaspoon paprika

1 (12-ounce) bag broccoli slaw

2 tablespoons white balsamic vinegar (or rice vinegar)

½ (16-ounce) package whole-wheat spaghetti

2 tablespoons chopped unsalted peanuts or almonds

1. Preheat the oven to 350°F.
2. Place the tofu between paper towels and set a heavy pot on top for about 5 minutes to remove the excess water.
3. In a 9-by-13-inch glass casserole dish, whisk together the olive oil, lime juice, garlic, honey, cumin, and paprika.
4. Cut the pressed tofu into cubes and add it to the marinade, stirring well to coat. Let marinate for at least 30 minutes.
5. Cook the spaghetti as directed on the package. (Don't add salt.)
6. Add the broccoli slaw and vinegar to the tofu, and stir to combine.
7. Bake in the preheated oven for 20 to 25 minutes. Serve over the spaghetti, topped with the nuts.

Substitution tip: For a more authentic version, use 100% buckwheat soba noodles instead of spaghetti. Bonus: Buckwheat soba noodles are gluten-free.

Veg-Out Ratatouille

1 POT | BUDGET-FRIENDLY | VEGAN

SERVES 4

PREP TIME:
15 MINUTES

COOK TIME:
40 MINUTES

Per serving
Calories: 183
Total Fat: 9g
Saturated Fat: 1g
Cholesterol: 0mg
Sodium: 90mg
Carbohydrates: 26g
Fiber: 9g
Protein: 5g

Ratatouille is a French vegetable stew that takes ordinary ingredients and makes them extraordinary. Tomatoes, eggplant, and zucchini are all high in blood pressure-controlling potassium. I like this dish over polenta, but you can also serve it as a side or as a topping for fish, chicken, or noodles. The flavors mingle overnight and become even more intense the next day.

2 tablespoons extra-virgin olive oil, divided, plus 1 teaspoon

1 medium eggplant, cut into 1-inch pieces

3 small zucchini, chopped

1 cup chopped onion

½ red bell pepper, chopped

3 garlic cloves, chopped

2 (14.5-ounce) cans low-sodium diced tomatoes

1 teaspoon dried thyme

1 teaspoon dried basil

1 teaspoon dried oregano

¼ teaspoon freshly ground black pepper

⅛ teaspoon red pepper flakes

1. Evenly brush the bottom and sides of a large skillet with 1 tablespoon of olive oil, and heat over low-medium heat.
2. Add the eggplant and cook for about 10 minutes, stirring often. Transfer to a plate and set aside.
3. Add 1 more tablespoon of oil along with the zucchini and onion, and sauté until softened but not brown, about 5 minutes. Stir in the bell pepper and garlic, and sauté 2 to 3 minutes more.
4. Add the sautéed eggplant, tomatoes, thyme, basil, oregano, black pepper, and red pepper flakes. Stir well and simmer over low heat for about 20 minutes.
5. Drizzle the remaining 1 teaspoon of oil on top before serving.

Storage tip: This dish will last one week in your refrigerator and freezes well for up to three months in an airtight container.

Bean-Chilada Casserole

BUDGET-FRIENDLY | GLUTEN-FREE | TIME-SAVER | VEGETARIAN

SERVES 4

PREP TIME:
15 MINUTES

COOK TIME:
25 MINUTES

Per serving
Calories: 411
Total Fat: 10g
Saturated Fat: 2g
Cholesterol: 5mg
Sodium: 285mg
Carbohydrates: 66g
Fiber: 15g
Protein: 21g

I often make this Mexican-inspired favorite because I love how the flavors meld in the oven. It's similar to a Mexican lasagna, so you can get your south-of-the-border food fix! This dish also freezes well, which makes it a great potluck item or food gift for friends or family.

1 (14.5-ounce) can low-sodium tomatoes (Mexican, fire-roasted, or diced)

1 (8-ounce) can low-sodium tomato sauce

½ cup salsa

2 (15.5-ounce) cans low-sodium black beans, drained and rinsed

¾ cup chopped onion

½ (4-ounce) can green chiles, drained but not rinsed

Cooking spray

6 to 8 small corn tortillas

4 tablespoons shredded low-fat Mexican-style cheese, divided

1 fresh avocado, chopped

½ cup nonfat plain Greek yogurt

1 teaspoon freshly squeezed lime juice

½ teaspoon ground cumin

½ teaspoon chili powder

1. Preheat the oven to 350°F.
2. In a medium bowl, combine the diced tomatoes, tomato sauce, and salsa.
3. In a separate medium bowl, combine the beans, onion, and green chiles.
4. Spray a 9-by-13-inch glass baking dish with cooking spray. Tear the small corn tortillas into quarters (roughly) and use about half the pieces to cover the bottom of the dish.
5. Layer half the bean mixture on top of the torn tortillas. Then layer half the tomato mixture over the beans. Sprinkle the whole dish with 2 tablespoons of cheese.
6. Repeat the process using the remaining torn tortilla pieces, remaining bean mixture, remaining tomato mixture, and remaining cheese.

7. Bake in the preheated oven for 25 minutes.
8. While it bakes, make the avocado sauce. In a small bowl, stir the avocado into the yogurt. Add the lime juice, cumin, and chili powder, and stir well. (The avocado should still be chunky.)
9. When the casserole is finished baking, let it cool slightly before serving so the layers hold together like lasagna. Serve topped with the avocado sauce.

Protein Pasta Pronto

BUDGET-FRIENDLY | GLUTEN-FREE | TIME-SAVER | VEGETARIAN

SERVES 4

PREP TIME:
15 MINUTES

COOK TIME:
25 MINUTES

Per serving
Calories: 242
Total Fat: 4g
Saturated Fat: <1g
Cholesterol: 0mg
Sodium: 191mg
Carbohydrates: 29g
Fiber: 11g
Protein: 14g

The herbaceous flavor of this pasta dish really hits the Italian spot! The protein boost comes from a high-protein pasta made with lentils instead of wheat. Since protein is such an important nutrient, especially in vegan and vegetarian dishes, this meal is a winner.

¾ cup lentil or chickpea fusilli or penne, such as Banza

2 teaspoons canola oil

½ sweet onion, chopped

3 garlic cloves, chopped

¼ teaspoon red pepper flakes

½ (14.5-ounce) can low-sodium diced tomatoes, with their juice

2 tablespoons low-sodium tomato paste

1½ teaspoons Italian seasoning

½ head fresh rainbow Swiss chard, chopped (including stems)

1 (15.5-ounce) can cannellini beans, drained and rinsed

¼ cup loosely packed fresh basil, chopped

1 teaspoon Parmesan cheese (optional)

1. Cook the pasta as directed on the package. (Don't add salt.) When draining, reserve the pasta water. Set the cooked pasta and reserved pasta water aside.

2. Evenly brush the bottom and sides of a large skillet with the oil. Add the onion and sauté over medium heat until soft, about 3 minutes. Then add the garlic and red pepper flakes, and cook for about 1 minute.

3. Reduce the heat to low, and add 1 cup of the reserved pasta water, diced tomatoes, tomato paste, and Italian seasoning. Stir until well blended.

4. Bring the heat back to medium and add the Swiss chard, cooking for 4 to 5 minutes, until the chard stalks are soft.

5. Add the cannellini beans and cooked pasta, stirring until everything is well combined and heated through, about 2 minutes.
6. Add a little more pasta water, if needed, and reduce the heat to a low simmer.
7. Just before serving, stir in the basil. Top with the Parmesan cheese (if using).

Recipe tip: Simply leave off the Parmesan to make this a protein-packed vegan dish.

Fiesta Taco Bowl

30 MINUTES | GLUTEN-FREE | TIME-SAVER | VEGETARIAN

SERVES 4

PREP TIME:
15 MINUTES

Per serving
Calories: 419
Total Fat: 19g
Saturated Fat: 3g
Cholesterol: 5mg
Sodium: 127mg
Carbohydrates: 53g
Fiber: 17g
Protein: 19g

Flavors of Mexico from the jalapeño, lime, and cilantro add interest and kick to this easy, quick salad. Mix some brown rice into the beans for a heavier meal, or just eat it as is for a low-calorie, high-nutrition lunch or dinner.

2 (15.5-ounce) cans low-sodium pinto beans, drained and rinsed

2 tablespoons chopped sweet onion

2 tablespoons salsa

2 tablespoons freshly squeezed lime juice, divided

2 teaspoons extra-virgin olive oil, plus 2 tablespoons

1½ teaspoons garlic powder

1½ teaspoons ground cumin

1 teaspoon seeded, finely chopped fresh jalapeño pepper

2 cups fresh baby spinach, cut into ribbons

1 cup coleslaw mix

¼ cup chopped fresh cilantro (optional)

½ cup chopped fresh tomatoes

½ cup nonfat plain Greek yogurt (or low-fat sour cream)

1 avocado, chopped

4 tablespoons low-fat shredded Cheddar or Mexican-style cheese

1. In a medium bowl, combine the pinto beans, onion, salsa, 1 tablespoon of lime juice, 2 teaspoons of olive oil, garlic powder, cumin, and jalapeño pepper.
2. In a separate medium bowl, combine the spinach, coleslaw mix, and cilantro (if using). Sprinkle with the remaining 1 tablespoon of lime juice and remaining 2 tablespoons of olive oil. Toss to coat.
3. Serve by plating the spinach salad first, then putting the bean mixture on top. (You can heat the bean mixture first if you want a warm salad.) Top with the tomatoes, yogurt, avocado, and shredded cheese, as desired.

Recipe tip: If you want tortilla chips with this dish, make your own without any salt. Cut whole-wheat or corn tortillas into fourths, brush with olive oil, and bake on a baking sheet at 450°F for 5 minutes.

Sweet Potato and Egg Hash with Shaved Brussels Sprouts

1 POT | BUDGET-FRIENDLY | VEGETARIAN

SERVES 3

PREP TIME:
10 MINUTES

COOK TIME:
35 MINUTES

Per serving
Calories: 284
Total Fat: 14g
Saturated Fat: 4g
Cholesterol: 285mg
Sodium: 138mg
Carbohydrates: 25g
Fiber: 4g
Protein: 13g

This sheet-pan dinner can also be eaten for breakfast, since the protein is eggs. The earthy flavors will wake up your taste buds. This hash is comfort food, no matter what time of day you choose to make it.

1 medium russet potato, peeled and cut into 1-inch cubes

1 large sweet potato, peeled and cut into 1-inch cubes

1 cup chopped onion

½ cup chopped red bell pepper

4 garlic cloves, chopped

1 tablespoon plus 1 teaspoon extra-virgin olive oil

2 cups shaved fresh Brussels sprouts

6 eggs

¼ cup low-fat shredded Swiss cheese

1. Preheat the oven to 425°F.
2. On a large baking sheet, spread out the russet potato, sweet potato, onion, bell pepper, and garlic. Add the olive oil and toss to coat.
3. Roast in the preheated oven for 15 minutes, then stir in the Brussels sprouts with the remaining 1 teaspoon of extra-virgin olive oil, and roast for an additional 10 minutes.
4. Remove the pan and make 6 wells in the vegetable mixture. Crack an egg into each well, then bake for 7 minutes more.
5. Remove to a cooling rack and sprinkle the Swiss cheese on top.

Ingredient tip: Swiss cheese is lower in salt and higher in protein and calcium than many other cheeses. Cream cheese, mozzarella, cottage cheese, ricotta, goat cheese, and Parmesan are also fairly low in sodium.

Zesty Vegan Lentil Sandwiches

VEGAN

SERVES 4

PREP TIME:
15 MINUTES

COOK TIME:
20 MINUTES

Per serving
Calories: 325
Total Fat: 7g
Saturated Fat: 1g
Cholesterol: 0mg
Sodium: 318mg
Carbohydrates: 58g
Fiber: 13g
Protein: 15g

This recipe can be doubled if you're serving a crowd. It also freezes beautifully, so put a batch in the freezer to thaw in a pinch on busy nights or for unexpected guests.

½ cup dried lentils

2 teaspoons canola oil

½ cup chopped yellow onion

½ cup chopped green bell pepper

½ cup chopped celery

½ cup grated carrots

2 large garlic cloves, finely chopped

3 ounces low-sodium tomato sauce

1 tablespoon tomato paste (no salt added)

1 heaping teaspoon chili powder

1 teaspoon dried oregano

1 teaspoon dried basil

½ teaspoon paprika

3 tablespoons water

2 tablespoons packed brown sugar

1 teaspoon dry mustard

4 whole-wheat buns (or hoagie rolls)

1. Wash the lentils in a sieve and remove any debris. Cook according to the package directions. Drain and set aside.
2. Evenly brush the bottom and sides of a skillet with the canola oil. Add the onion, bell pepper, celery, and carrots, and sauté over medium heat until soft, 3 to 4 minutes. Stir in the garlic and sauté for 1 minute more.
3. Stir the cooked lentils into this mixture, followed by the tomato sauce, tomato paste, chili powder, oregano, basil, and paprika. Then stir in the water, brown sugar, and dry mustard, and cook for 10 minutes.
4. Turn off the heat and let sit for 3 minutes to thicken. Serve on the whole-wheat buns.

Rainbow Corn and Bean Salad

GLUTEN-FREE | TIME-SAVER | VEGAN

SERVES 5

PREP TIME:
20 MINUTES,
PLUS 2 TO
4 HOURS TO
CHILL

Per serving
Calories: 235
Total Fat: 12g
Saturated Fat: 2g
Cholesterol: 0mg
Sodium: 12mg
Carbohydrates: 27g
Fiber: 6g
Protein: 7g

This rainbow-colored, no-cook bean salad can be served over greens for a refreshing lunch, as a dip for homemade tortilla chips, or as a filling for a whole-wheat tortilla or wrap. It's also a great side for any meal or potluck. Quick and convenient, it uses low-salt canned products along with a few fresh ones to deliver crunch and pizzazz.

¼ cup freshly squeezed lime juice (from 1 to 2 limes)

¼ cup extra-virgin olive oil

¼ cup chopped fresh cilantro

½ teaspoon chili powder

Pinch cayenne pepper

1 (15.5-ounce) can low-sodium black beans, drained and rinsed

1 (15.5-ounce) can low-sodium corn, drained and rinsed

½ cup shredded purple cabbage

½ cup chopped red bell pepper

½ cup chopped green bell pepper

¼ cup chopped scallions

½ small jalapeño or serrano pepper, cored, seeded, and finely chopped

1. In a small bowl, whisk together the lime juice, olive oil, cilantro, chili powder, and cayenne to make the dressing.
2. In a separate medium bowl, combine the black beans, corn, cabbage, red bell pepper, green bell pepper, scallions, and jalapeño pepper.
3. Add the dressing to the bean salad and stir well. Refrigerate for 2 to 4 hours before serving.

Ingredient tip: When touching jalapeño peppers (or any other hot pepper), always use some kind of rubber or plastic gloves to protect yourself from capsaicin, the burning natural chemical they contain. It doesn't come off your hands easily, and if it gets in your eyes, it'll hurt.

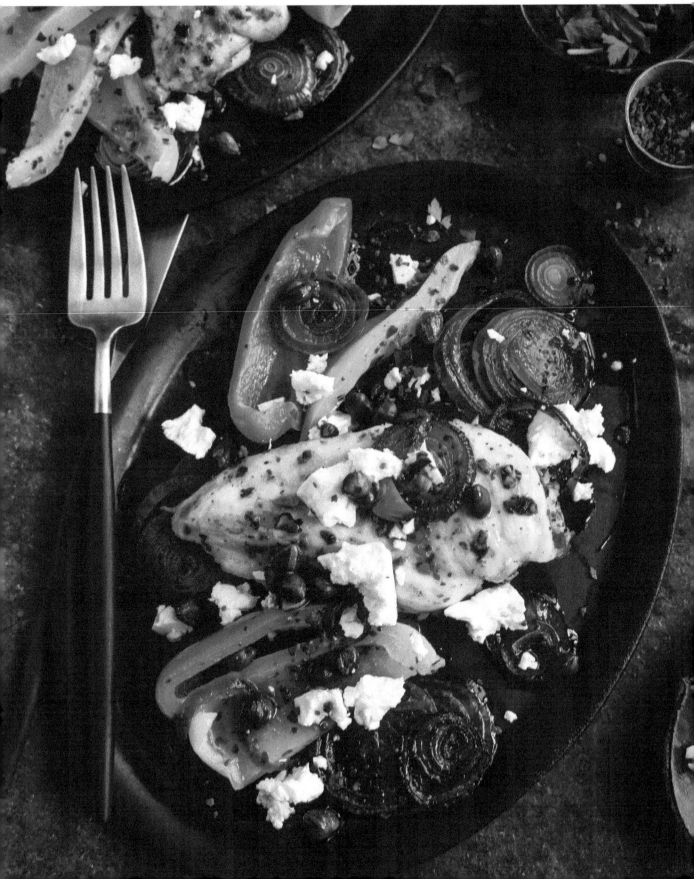

chapter seven

SEAFOOD AND POULTRY MAINS

◀ Garlic Chicken with Peppers and Feta Cheese, _page 110_

Tomato, Mozzarella, and Basil Chicken

GLUTEN-FREE

SERVES 4

PREP TIME:
15 MINUTES,
PLUS 4 HOURS
TO MARINATE

COOK TIME:
15 MINUTES

Per serving
Calories: 286
Total Fat: 15g
Saturated Fat: 3g
Cholesterol: 73mg
Sodium: 291mg
Carbohydrates: 9g
Fiber: 1g
Protein: 28g

This recipe is a workhorse in terms of versatility. The leftovers can be turned into many different meals. Try using them in hot or cold pasta dishes, sandwiches, or salads. You may want to double the recipe so you can repurpose the extra chicken for more meals later in the week.

¼ cup white wine

2 tablespoons chopped shallot

2 tablespoons extra-virgin olive oil

1 tablespoon freshly squeezed lemon juice

2 teaspoons honey

1 teaspoon fresh lemon zest

½ teaspoon Dijon mustard

½ teaspoon dried thyme

½ teaspoon chopped fresh rosemary leaves

4 boneless, skinless chicken breasts

2 teaspoons canola oil

1 cup fresh whole basil leaves

4 or 5 small tomatoes, sliced

½ cup shredded part-skim mozzarella cheese

1. In a small bowl, whisk together the white wine, shallot, olive oil, lemon juice, honey, lemon zest, mustard, thyme, and rosemary.
2. Pat the chicken breasts dry with paper towels and put them in a leakproof sealable bag. Pour the marinade over the chicken, seal the bag, and refrigerate for at least 4 hours, turning the bag after 2 hours.
3. Remove the marinated chicken from the refrigerator, drain it (discard the marinade), and pat the chicken dry with paper towels.

4. Evenly brush the bottom and sides of a medium sauté pan with the canola oil. Cook the chicken breasts, covered, over medium heat, for 5 to 6 minutes, then turn them over and continue to cook for another 5 minutes, until they're no longer pink inside.

5. Place a few basil leaves on top of each chicken breast, followed by a few of the sliced tomatoes. Top with equal amounts of shredded mozzarella cheese. Cover and let cook on low heat for about 1 minute more to melt the cheese. Spoon juices from the pan over the chicken when serving.

Maple-Spice Chicken with Vegetables

BUDGET-FRIENDLY | TIME-SAVER

SERVES 4

PREP TIME:
10 MINUTES,
PLUS AT LEAST
4 HOURS TO
MARINATE

COOK TIME:
20 MINUTES

Per serving
Calories: 337
Total Fat: 21g
Saturated Fat: 4g
Cholesterol: 90mg
Sodium: 222mg
Carbohydrates: 21g
Fiber: 3g
Protein: 18g

Baking-sheet dinners save time in the kitchen, because you can cook the meat and vegetables together in one pan. This recipe requires marinating both the chicken and the vegetables, but if you prep ahead of time, you can just dump the ingredients onto the pan when you get home, and you'll have a full meal on the table in 20 minutes. Your entire family will like this chicken dish—even kids and grandkids!

¼ cup extra-virgin olive oil

¼ cup apple-cider vinegar

3 tablespoons maple syrup

1 tablespoon garlic powder

½ teaspoon ground ginger

½ teaspoon ground allspice

½ teaspoon dried thyme

⅛ teaspoon cayenne pepper

1 (12-ounce) bag mixed broccoli and cauliflower florets

4 large carrots, peeled and cut into coins

10 to 12 boneless, skinless chicken thighs

Cooking spray

1. In a small bowl, whisk together the olive oil, vinegar, maple syrup, garlic powder, ginger, allspice, thyme, and cayenne pepper. Divide this marinade in half between two 1-gallon leakproof sealable plastic bags.
2. Cut the broccoli and cauliflower florets into equal sizes, if necessary. Put the broccoli, cauliflower, and carrots in one of the marinade bags.
3. Pat the chicken thighs dry and put them in the other marinade bag.
4. Seal both bags and refrigerate overnight or for at least 4 hours, turning the bags once.
5. Preheat the oven to 425°F.

6. Coat a baking sheet with cooking spray and spread the vegetables on it. Place the chicken thighs on top of the vegetables. Roast for 15 to 20 minutes, until the vegetables are tender-crisp.

Ingredient tip: The bags of precut produce are simply a shortcut. Feel free to chop your own broccoli and cauliflower to cut costs even further.

White Wine Chicken Scampi

30 MINUTES

SERVES 4

PREP TIME:
15 MINUTES

COOK TIME:
15 MINUTES

Per serving
Calories: 363
Total Fat: 8g
Saturated Fat: 1g
Cholesterol: 51mg
Sodium: 216mg
Carbohydrates: 51g
Fiber: 10g
Protein: 27g

Yes, you can eat pasta if you have high blood pressure—as long as you limit the salt. First, skip salting the pasta water. Second, use very small amounts of Parmesan cheese, just enough to enhance flavor. You'll be helping your blood pressure by keeping the sodium low in this delicious meal.

8 ounces whole-wheat linguine or spaghetti

3 teaspoons extra-virgin olive oil, divided

1 large shallot, finely chopped

2 large boneless, skinless chicken breasts, cut into 1-by-3-inch pieces

3 large garlic cloves, chopped

⅛ teaspoon red pepper flakes

½ cup white wine

½ cup low-sodium chicken broth

3 tablespoons freshly squeezed lemon juice, divided

1 (14.5-ounce) can artichoke hearts, drained, rinsed, and quartered

½ cup chopped zucchini

1 teaspoon Italian seasoning

1 teaspoon fresh lemon zest

2 tablespoons Parmesan cheese

1. Cook the linguine according to the package directions (don't add salt). Drain the pasta and reserve 4 tablespoons of the pasta water.
2. Evenly brush a large skillet with 2 teaspoons of olive oil. Add the shallot and sauté over medium heat until soft and almost translucent, about 5 minutes. Add the chicken pieces and sauté for another 3 to 4 minutes. Add the garlic and red pepper flakes and stir until fragrant, about 1 minute.
3. Add 2 tablespoons of the reserved pasta water, the wine, broth, and 2 tablespoons of lemon juice. Cook until the chicken is fork-tender, 2 to 3 minutes more. Remove the chicken to a warm plate.

4. To the skillet, add the artichoke hearts, zucchini, Italian seasoning, and remaining 1 teaspoon of olive oil. Cook, covered, for 2 minutes, stirring often.
5. Add the chicken back to the pan. Add 2 more tablespoons of the pasta water, the remaining 1 tablespoon of lemon juice, and the lemon zest. Stir to combine.
6. Transfer the chicken mixture to a large bowl. Add the cooked linguine and Parmesan cheese, tossing well to combine before serving.

Ingredient tip: If you skip salting the pasta water, you can use it to thicken sauces and make them creamier without adding fat or salt.

Fish Wraps with Sriracha Slaw

30 MINUTES | BUDGET-FRIENDLY | TIME-SAVER

SERVES 4

PREP TIME:
15 MINUTES

COOK TIME:
10 MINUTES

Per serving
Calories: 320
Total Fat: 8g
Saturated Fat: 1g
Cholesterol: 13mg
Sodium: 380mg
Carbohydrates: 34g
Fiber: 9g
Protein: 28g

This lively recipe has a creamy, piquant (but not fiery hot) sauce that's the perfect addition to the mild fish. Fish adds potassium and other important nutrients to our diet, so getting in two to three servings of fish every week is great for lowering blood pressure. This simple dish is a superb light lunch or dinner, especially with the refreshing slaw.

FOR THE SLAW

¼ cup nonfat plain Greek yogurt

¼ cup low-fat mayonnaise

1 tablespoon freshly squeezed lime juice

1 teaspoon sriracha sauce (or more if desired)

1 teaspoon finely chopped red onion

½ teaspoon garlic powder

½ teaspoon ground cumin

½ (10-ounce) bag shredded Brussels sprouts

2 cups store-bought coleslaw mix

¼ cup chopped scallions

¼ cup chopped fresh cilantro (optional)

FOR THE FISH WRAPS

Nonstick cooking spray

16 ounces cod (or any white fish), cut into 4 pieces

1 cup flour, in a shallow bowl for dredging

2 teaspoons garlic powder

2 teaspoons ground cumin

2 teaspoons smoked paprika

4 (5- to 6-inch) whole-wheat tortillas

2 limes, quartered

1 avocado, finely chopped

To make the slaw

1. In a large bowl, whisk together the Greek yogurt, mayonnaise, lime juice, sriracha, onion, garlic powder, and cumin.
2. Add the shredded Brussels sprouts, coleslaw mix, scallions, and cilantro (if using), and toss to coat.

To make the fish wraps

1. Heat the oven to 425°F. Spray a baking sheet with nonstick cooking spray.
2. Dredge each piece of fish in flour, on both sides. Sprinkle each side with garlic powder, cumin, and smoked paprika.
3. Put the fish on the prepared pan and bake in the preheated oven for 8 to 10 minutes, depending on the thickness of your fish fillets (about 10 minutes per inch of thickness).
4. Wrap the tortillas in a paper towel and microwave for about 15 seconds until warm.
5. Spread ½ cup of the sriracha slaw evenly on each tortilla and place the fish on top. Squeeze juice from the lime wedges over the fish and sprinkle with the avocado. Roll up the tortillas and enjoy!

Salmon with Glazed Peach Sauce and Black Rice

30 MINUTES | BUDGET-FRIENDLY | GLUTEN-FREE | TIME-SAVER

SERVES 4

PREP TIME:
10 MINUTES

COOK TIME:
15 MINUTES

Per serving
Calories: 442
Total Fat: 16g
Saturated Fat: 5g
Cholesterol: 46mg
Sodium: 162mg
Carbohydrates: 47g
Fiber: 4g
Protein: 25g

The elegant, fruity, and easy-to-make sauce in this dish plays off the richness of the salmon and enhances it with a little natural sweetness. This whole recipe takes just minutes to prepare. Feel free to grill or pan-sauté the salmon if you prefer not to turn on the oven. This dish is breathtakingly colorful served over black rice—but if you don't have any made, and you're pressed for time, any rice will be delicious.

FOR THE PEACH SAUCE

1 (14.5-ounce) can sliced peaches in their own juice (no sugar added)

2 teaspoons extra-virgin olive oil, divided

2 tablespoons finely chopped red onion

1 tablespoon peach jam

1 tablespoon white balsamic vinegar

1 teaspoon seeded, chopped jalapeño pepper (optional)

½ teaspoon Dijon mustard

FOR THE SALMON

1 tablespoon peach jam

1 tablespoon Dijon mustard

2 teaspoons white balsamic vinegar

1 teaspoon extra-virgin olive oil

1 pound salmon fillet (preferably wild-caught)

¼ cup chopped fresh cilantro, for garnish, if desired

3 cups cooked black rice

To make the peach sauce

1. Strain the can of peaches, reserving the juice. Finely chop half the peaches. Save the other half of the peaches for another recipe or to eat as a snack.
2. Evenly brush the bottom and sides of a small sauté pan with 1 teaspoon of olive oil. Over low heat, sauté the red onion for 1 to 2 minutes, making sure not to brown it.

3. Add half the reserved peach juice to the pan. Then add the peach jam, vinegar, jalapeño pepper (if using), Dijon mustard, and the remaining 1 teaspoon of olive oil. Whisk all the ingredients together.

4. Heat to bubbling and cook for 2 to 3 minutes, until thickened. Remove from the heat and stir in the chopped peaches. If the sauce is too thick, whisk in a bit more reserved peach juice. Keep warm.

To make the salmon

1. Preheat the oven to 425°F. Line a baking sheet with aluminum foil.

2. In a small bowl, whisk together the peach jam, Dijon mustard, vinegar, and olive oil.

3. Pat the salmon fillet dry and spread the jam mixture evenly on top. Bake on the prepared baking sheet in the preheated oven for 10 to 14 minutes, depending on the thickness of the fillet (about 10 minutes per inch of thickness).

4. Cut the fillet into 4 equal pieces. Spoon the sauce over each piece and sprinkle with the cilantro, if desired. Serve over the black rice.

Cooking tip: Remove the fish from the oven a few minutes before you think it's done—fish continues to cook after you remove it from heat!

Chicken Curry in a Hurry

1 POT | 30 MINUTES

SERVES 4

PREP TIME:
15 MINUTES

COOK TIME:
15 MINUTES

Per serving
Calories: 423
Total Fat: 12g
Saturated Fat: 6g
Cholesterol: 65mg
Sodium: 265mg
Carbohydrates: 49g
Fiber: 6g
Protein: 29g

Curry is a mixture of potent spices that adds a strong and distinct aroma to any dish. The creamy coconut-milk sauce of this recipe coats the mouthwatering chicken pieces and delivers exquisite flavor. This dish also adds more veggies to your day to help lower your blood pressure. Serve it over brown rice for extra fiber.

1 pound boneless, skinless chicken breasts, cut into 2-inch cubes

1 tablespoon flour

1 tablespoon curry powder, plus 1 teaspoon

⅛ teaspoon freshly ground black pepper

2 teaspoons canola oil

1 (14-ounce) can light coconut milk

1 tablespoon packed brown sugar

1 teaspoon garlic powder

1 teaspoon onion powder

¼ teaspoon cayenne pepper

1 (10-ounce) bag mixed broccoli and cauliflower florets

1 cup grated carrots

¼ cup raisins (optional)

3 cups cooked brown rice

1. In a large, sealable bag, combine the chicken cubes, flour, 1 tablespoon of curry powder, and black pepper. Shake to coat.
2. Evenly brush the bottom and sides of a large skillet with the canola oil. Sauté the chicken over medium heat for 5 minutes, stirring frequently to cook all sides.
3. Add the remaining 1 teaspoon of curry powder, coconut milk, brown sugar, garlic powder, onion powder, and cayenne. Stir well. Add the broccoli and cauliflower florets and carrots, stirring until combined. Simmer on low for 10 minutes until thick, adding a little water, if necessary, to reach your desired thickness.
4. Top with the raisins (if using), and serve over the brown rice.

Halibut with Roasted Tomato and Basil Sauce

30 MINUTES | GLUTEN-FREE

SERVES 4

PREP TIME:
20 MINUTES

COOK TIME:
10 MINUTES

Per serving
Calories: 299
Total Fat: 17g
Saturated Fat: 2g
Cholesterol: 47mg
Sodium: 90mg
Carbohydrates: 7g
Fiber: 1g
Protein: 31g

If you're a tomato fan like me, you'll love this ruby-red tomato sauce that cooks right in the pan along with the fish. So easy, yet sophisticated! I like this fish served with a wild rice pilaf to add whole grains. Many of the store-bought pilaf mixtures are high in salt, however, so look for a brand such as Lundberg that has no added salt.

1 pound ripe fresh tomatoes, chopped, with their juices (do not use Roma tomatoes)

¼ cup chopped fresh basil

3 tablespoons extra-virgin olive oil, plus 2 teaspoons

3 garlic cloves, chopped

1 tablespoon balsamic vinegar

Pinch cayenne pepper

4 halibut (or other white fish) fillets, about 4 ounces each

Fresh parsley, for garnish

1. Preheat the oven to 400°F.
2. In a medium bowl, stir together the tomatoes (and their juices), basil, 3 tablespoons of olive oil, garlic, vinegar, and cayenne. Let sit.
3. Brush the bottom of an oven-safe skillet or sauté pan with the remaining 2 teaspoons of oil. Pat the fish dry and place in the pan. Cook for 3 minutes over medium heat, then flip. Spread the tomato mixture around the fish.
4. Bake, uncovered, in the preheated oven for 5 minutes.
5. Garnish with the parsley and serve.

One-Pan Herb-Roasted Chicken with Caramelized Shallots

1 POT

SERVES 6 TO 8

PREP TIME:
25 MINUTES

COOK TIME:
1 HOUR

Per serving
Calories: 303
Total Fat: 8g
Saturated Fat: 1g
Cholesterol: 49mg
Sodium: 53mg
Carbohydrates: 28g
Fiber: 2g
Protein: 21g

This heavenly whole-roasted chicken will fill your home with a wonderful herbaceous scent as it bakes. Just imagine how all those caramelized shallots and garlic will taste. You won't be disappointed! The rich "broth" made from the chicken drippings is perfect for dipping bread or as a delectable sauce for the vegetables alongside the chicken.

1 whole (5-pound) roasting chicken, rinsed

3 tablespoons freshly squeezed lemon juice, divided (reserve the lemon rind)

3 teaspoons dried thyme, divided

Cooking spray

2 tablespoons extra-virgin olive oil

1 teaspoon garlic powder

1½ pounds baby potatoes

14 shallots, peeled and left whole

½ (5-ounce) bag baby carrots

6 garlic cloves, peeled and left whole

1½ cups dry white wine

1 teaspoon dried sage

1 teaspoon dried rosemary

1. Preheat the oven to 400°F.
2. Remove the giblets and gizzards from the chicken, and pat dry. Rub the inside of the chicken cavity with 1 tablespoon of lemon juice and the lemon rind. Cut the lemon rind into four pieces and use it to stuff the cavity. Sprinkle the cavity with 1 teaspoon of thyme.
3. Spray a large, shallow roasting pan with cooking spray, and put the chicken on it, breast-side up. Rub the outside of the chicken with the olive oil and season it by sprinkling it with the garlic powder and 1 teaspoon of thyme. Roast in the preheated oven for 15 minutes.

4. Remove the pan from the oven and add the potatoes, shallots, carrots, and garlic, spreading them around the chicken in the pan. Pour the wine over everything, along with the remaining 2 tablespoons of lemon juice. Sprinkle the sage, rosemary, and remaining 1 teaspoon of thyme over the entire pan.
5. Roast, uncovered, for another 45 minutes, stirring the veggies at least once, until the juices from the chicken run clear and a food thermometer inserted into the chicken reads 165°F.

Recipe tip: Feel free to substitute 1 tablespoon of fresh herbs for each teaspoon of dried herbs in this recipe.

Garlic Chicken with Peppers and Feta Cheese

BUDGET-FRIENDLY

SERVES 4

PREP TIME:
15 MINUTES,
PLUS AT LEAST
6 HOURS TO
MARINATE

COOK TIME:
40 MINUTES

Per serving
Calories: 350
Total Fat: 24g
Saturated Fat: 4g
Cholesterol: 71mg
Sodium: 308mg
Carbohydrates: 13g
Fiber: 3g
Protein: 26g

This lean, nutrient-packed dish creates a flavorful sauce while baking in the oven. It's perfect for serving over brown rice or whole-wheat pasta. If you're not fond of peppers, simply substitute your favorite vegetables.

5 tablespoons freshly squeezed lemon juice (from 2 to 3 lemons), divided

5 tablespoons plus 2 teaspoons extra-virgin olive oil, divided

3 garlic cloves, chopped

1 teaspoon dried oregano, divided

⅛ teaspoon red pepper flakes

4 medium boneless, skinless chicken breasts

3 bell peppers (red, orange, or yellow), seeded and cut into ½-inch strips

1 cup sliced onion rounds

2 tablespoons feta cheese

2 tablespoons capers, drained and rinsed

1 tablespoon chopped fresh or dried parsley (optional)

1. In a small bowl, whisk together 4 tablespoons of lemon juice, 3 tablespoons of olive oil, the garlic, ½ teaspoon of oregano, and the red pepper flakes.
2. Pat the chicken breasts dry and pound them to an even thickness between two sheets of waxed paper.
3. Place the chicken in a leakproof plastic bag and pour the marinade over them. Marinate, refrigerated, for at least 6 hours.
4. Preheat the oven to 400°F.
5. Spread the bell peppers and onions out on a large baking pan. Drizzle with 1 tablespoon of olive oil followed by the remaining ½ teaspoon of oregano.

6. Evenly brush a large skillet with 2 teaspoons of olive oil. Place the chicken in the skillet and brown over medium heat, about 4 minutes each side. When browned, put the chicken breasts on top of the pepper and onion mixture in the baking pan. Drizzle the entire pan with the remaining 1 tablespoon of lemon juice and 1 tablespoon of olive oil.

7. Cover the pan tightly with aluminum foil, and bake in the preheated oven for about 30 minutes. Use a food thermometer to be sure the chicken reaches 165°F.

8. Sprinkle the entire dish with the feta, capers, and parsley (if using) before serving.

Fresh Tomato and Shrimp Spaghetti

1 POT

SERVES 5

PREP TIME:
15 MINUTES

COOK TIME:
20 MINUTES

Per serving
Calories: 391
Total Fat: 10g
Saturated Fat: 2g
Cholesterol: 139mg
Sodium: 169mg
Carbohydrates: 45g
Fiber: 7g
Protein: 26g

This easy shrimp sauté makes its own complex sauce from the mingling of the wine and the juices from the shrimp. The not-to-be-missed sauce combined with tomatoes, peppers, and onions will make peeling those shrimp totally worthwhile! Add a side salad and dinner's ready!

1 (8-ounce) package whole-wheat spaghetti

1 pound frozen raw shrimp, thawed (wild or USA-farmed, if possible)

2 tablespoons extra-virgin olive oil, plus 1 teaspoon

4 garlic cloves, minced

¼ teaspoon red pepper flakes

1 cup chopped red onion

½ cup chopped red bell pepper

1½ pounds fresh tomatoes, finely chopped (including the juices)

½ cup dry white wine (such as sauvignon blanc)

1 teaspoon dried basil

1 teaspoon dried oregano

¼ teaspoon freshly ground black pepper

1 to 2 tablespoons Parmesan cheese

2 tablespoons chopped fresh parsley, for garnish

1. Cook the spaghetti according to the package directions. (Do not add salt.)
2. If necessary (check the package), peel, devein, and remove the tails from the shrimp.
3. Evenly brush the bottom and sides of a large skillet with 2 tablespoons of olive oil. Add the shrimp, garlic, and red pepper flakes, and sauté over low-medium heat, stirring often, for about 2 minutes. Do not overcook. Remove the mixture from the pan and set aside.

4. Add the remaining 1 teaspoon of olive oil to the pan. Add the onion and bell pepper, and sauté for 2 to 3 minutes. Stir in the tomatoes, white wine, basil, oregano, and black pepper. Simmer, uncovered, for about 15 minutes.

5. Reduce the heat to low and add the shrimp back to the pan. Stir gently to mix into the thickened sauce. Sprinkle the sauce with the Parmesan cheese before serving over the spaghetti. Garnish each serving with parsley.

Sweet-and-Savory Chicken over Couscous

BUDGET-FRIENDLY | TIME-SAVER

SERVES 4

PREP TIME:
15 MINUTES

COOK TIME:
20 MINUTES

Per serving
Calories: 457
Total Fat: 16g
Saturated Fat: 3g
Cholesterol: 90mg
Sodium: 196mg
Carbohydrates: 54g
Fiber: 6g
Protein: 26g

This fast skillet dish accentuates both sweet and savory tastes from Middle Eastern cuisine. The pungent flavors of spices, dried fruit, and nuts will excite your taste buds. I've used whole-wheat couscous here, but this is also wonderful served over quinoa. Add a green salad to create an interesting and delicious meal!

1 (14.5-ounce) can crushed tomatoes, with their juice (no salt added)

½ (8-ounce) can tomato sauce (no salt added)

2 tablespoons chopped canned green chiles, drained and rinsed

2 tablespoons Craisins (or golden raisins)

1 tablespoon maple syrup

¾ teaspoon ground cumin

½ teaspoon ground cinnamon

½ teaspoon ground coriander

⅛ teaspoon freshly ground black pepper

2 teaspoons extra-virgin olive oil

10 to 12 boneless, skinless chicken thighs

½ cup chopped sweet onion

3 garlic cloves, chopped

¼ cup toasted unsalted almonds

4 cups cooked whole-wheat couscous

1. In a large bowl, combine the crushed tomatoes, tomato sauce, green chiles, Craisins, maple syrup, cumin, cinnamon, coriander, and black pepper.

2. Evenly brush the bottom and sides of a pan with the olive oil. Pat the chicken thighs dry with a paper towel. Add the chicken thighs and the onion to the pan. Cook over medium heat for 4 to 5 minutes per side. During the last minute of the second side, add the garlic and stir.

3. Add the tomato mixture to the pan and stir it in with the chicken. Cover the pan and simmer on low for about 10 minutes, adding a little water if the sauce gets too thick.
4. Remove from the heat and stir in the almonds. Serve over the couscous.

Substitution tip: Make this dish vegan by skipping the chicken and adding a can of low-sodium chickpeas, drained and rinsed, to the tomato mixture.

Anytime Tuna Patties

30 MINUTES

SERVES 4

PREP TIME:
10 TO
15 MINUTES

COOK TIME:
LESS THAN
5 MINUTES

Per serving
Calories: 106
Total Fat: 5g
Saturated Fat: 1g
Cholesterol: 60mg
Sodium: 147mg
Carbohydrates: 6g
Fiber: <1g
Protein: 10g

Stumped for a quick dinner idea? This recipe is your answer, and you can be assured it brings canned tuna to a new level! It's so flavorful it doesn't even need a sauce, and it goes great alongside your favorite rice pilaf or my Garlic Roasted Red Potatoes (page 64). Dinner: done!

1 (6-ounce) can tuna (white albacore or skipjack, packed in water, no salt added)

2 tablespoons finely chopped fresh basil

2 tablespoons finely chopped red bell pepper

2 tablespoons finely chopped scallion

2 tablespoons finely chopped celery

¼ cup plain panko crumbs

1 egg, whisked

1 teaspoon fresh lemon zest

½ teaspoon freshly squeezed lemon juice

½ teaspoon Dijon mustard

2 teaspoons extra-virgin olive oil

1 teaspoon garlic powder

1 tablespoon sriracha mayonnaise (optional)

1. Drain the tuna and use a fork to flake it into a mixing bowl.
2. Add the basil, bell pepper, scallion, and celery to the tuna. Then add the panko crumbs, egg, lemon zest, lemon juice, and mustard. Mix thoroughly to combine.
3. Form the tuna mixture into 3-inch-wide patties.
4. Evenly brush the bottom and sides of a sauté pan with the olive oil and sauté the patties on low-medium heat for about 2 minutes each side, until lightly browned.
5. Drizzle the sriracha mayonnaise (if using) on top, and serve.

Lemon-Pepper Baked Chicken

BUDGET-FRIENDLY

SERVES 4

PREP TIME:
10 MINUTES

COOK TIME:
1 HOUR

Per serving
Calories: 291
Total Fat: 7g
Saturated Fat: 1g
Cholesterol: 185mg
Sodium: 175mg
Carbohydrates: 21g
Fiber: <1g
Protein: 33g

Baking is an easy way to prepare chicken: You can put it in the oven and prepare the rest of the meal while it's cooking. This dish is exceptionally juicy because it uses bone-in split chicken breasts, and the moisture is locked in with a full-flavor (but low-salt) seasoned coating. The outside gets crispy while the inside stays fork-tender.

2 eggs, beaten

½ cup low-fat or skim milk

1 tablespoon fresh lemon zest

1 tablespoon freshly squeezed lemon juice

½ teaspoon garlic powder

4 bone-in split chicken breasts, skins removed

1 cup plain panko crumbs, in a shallow bowl for dredging

4 teaspoons Mrs. Dash Lemon Pepper (with no salt)

2 tablespoons extra-virgin olive oil

1. Preheat the oven to 350°F. Prepare a baking pan by lining it with nonstick aluminum foil.
2. In a large bowl, whisk together the eggs, milk, lemon zest, lemon juice, and garlic powder. Set aside.
3. Remove any fatty attachments on the chicken and pat it dry. Dip each chicken piece into the egg mixture, completely immersing it, and then immediately press it into the panko. Repeat on each side of the chicken.
4. Place the chicken breasts on the baking pan. Sprinkle each breast with the lemon pepper.
5. Bake the chicken in the preheated oven for 45 minutes, then remove and drizzle each chicken breast with the olive oil. Put the chicken back in the oven and bake for 15 more minutes, or until the coating browns and gets crispy.

Ingredient tip: Read the label when buying lemon-pepper seasoning—most are loaded with salt! I recommend Mrs. Dash brand, which has no salt.

Mediterranean Cod Purses

30 MINUTES | GLUTEN-FREE

SERVES 4

PREP TIME:
15 MINUTES

COOK TIME:
15 MINUTES

Per serving
Calories: 209
Total Fat: 7g
Saturated Fat: 1g
Cholesterol: 62mg
Sodium: 229mg
Carbohydrates: 10g
Fiber: 3g
Protein: 27g

This recipe looks and sounds fancy, but it's a cinch to prepare. It uses a French cooking method called en papillote *(literally "in paper"), in which a sealed "purse" of parchment paper or aluminum foil locks in the flavor and moisture as it steams the fish and vegetables. The result is a silky, flaky fish, an appetizing juice, and easy kitchen cleanup.*

1 medium zucchini, cut into matchsticks

1 small yellow squash, cut into matchsticks

½ small white onion, sliced

¾ cup halved grape tomatoes

1½ tablespoons extra-virgin olive oil

¼ teaspoon freshly ground black pepper

¼ teaspoon red pepper flakes (optional)

4 pieces of cod (or any white fish), 4 to 6 ounces each

2 teaspoons garlic powder, divided

2 teaspoons dried thyme, divided

2 tablespoons capers, drained and rinsed, divided

1 lemon, cut into thin slices

4 tablespoons white wine, divided

1. Preheat the oven to 425°F.
2. In a mixing bowl, toss the zucchini, yellow squash, onion, and tomatoes with the olive oil, black pepper, and red pepper flakes (if using).
3. Pat the fish dry and sprinkle each piece with ¼ teaspoon of the garlic powder and ¼ teaspoon of dried thyme.
4. To assemble the purses, divide the vegetable mixture into four, and lay each portion in the center of a 12-by-12-inch piece of aluminum foil. Place one piece of fish, seasoning-side down, lengthwise on each mound of vegetables so it fits nicely on top. Now that the unseasoned side of the fish is showing, sprinkle each piece with another ¼ teaspoon of the garlic powder and ¼ teaspoon of thyme.

5. Sprinkle ½ tablespoon of the capers on top of each fish-and-vege-table mound. Add 2 or 3 slices of lemon and 1 tablespoon of white wine to each.

6. To seal the purses, pull the top and bottom foil edges up and over the fish. Bring the edges together and make 2 to 3 small folds, rolling them down, and pinching them tightly—it will look like a tent. Now fold the sides in toward the center of the fish, repeat the folding, and pinch them off. Be sure the purses are sealed tightly.

7. Place on a baking sheet and bake in the preheated oven for 12 minutes. Remove and let stand a few minutes before serving. Be careful: Steam will escape when opening the pouches!

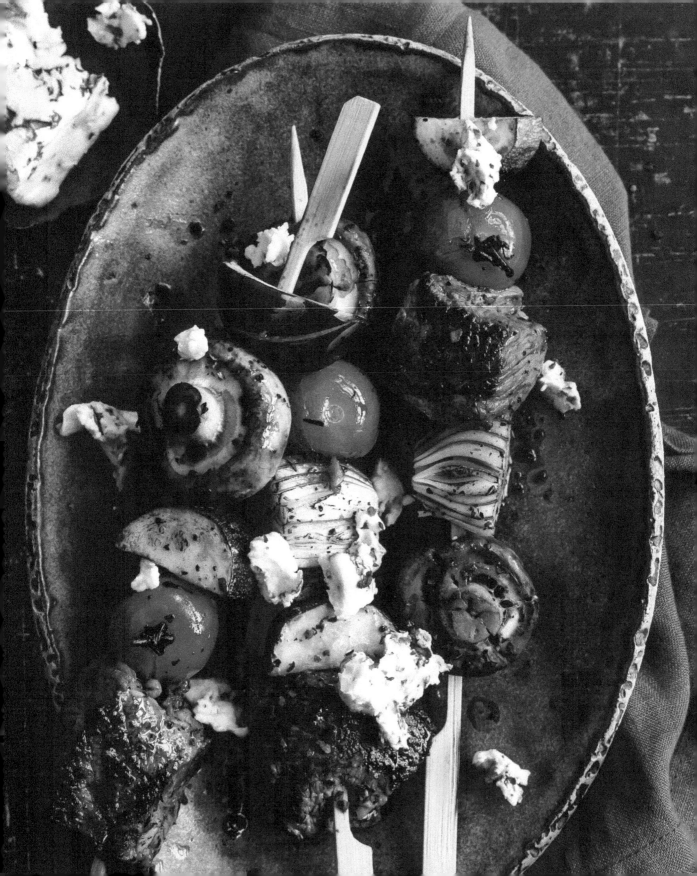

chapter eight

BEEF AND PORK MAINS

Grilled Steak with Roasted Onions and Peppers

BUDGET FRIENDLY | GLUTEN-FREE

SERVES 4

PREP TIME:
10 MINUTES,
PLUS
OVERNIGHT TO
MARINATE

COOK TIME:
35 MINUTES

Per serving
Calories: 407
Total Fat: 32g
Saturated Fat: 8g
Cholesterol: 65mg
Sodium: 63mg
Carbohydrates: 7g
Fiber: 2g
Protein: 22g

This is a budget-friendly recipe for a small group that can be easily sized up for a crowd. Marinating less tender cuts of beef, like the one recommended here, is a great way to bring out their flavor so you can enjoy them as much as the more tender cuts of beef that are twice the price.

FOR THE STEAK

¼ cup extra-virgin olive oil

2 tablespoons red-wine vinegar

1 teaspoon dried basil

¼ teaspoon red pepper flakes

4 sirloin tip steaks

FOR THE VEGETABLES

1 large sweet onion, sliced

1½ tablespoons extra-virgin olive oil, divided

2 red bell peppers, cored, seeded, and halved

To marinate the steak

1. In a small mixing bowl, whisk together the olive oil, vinegar, dried basil, and red pepper flakes to make the marinade.
2. Place the steaks in a nonreactive sealable container or a leakproof plastic bag. Seal the container and marinate in the refrigerator overnight or longer.

To cook the vegetables and steak

1. Preheat the oven to 450°F.
2. Toss the onion with 1 tablespoon of olive oil to coat well, then spread the mixture out on one side of a baking pan.
3. Use the remaining ½ tablespoon of olive oil to rub the outsides of the peppers with oil, and then place them cut-side down on the other side of the baking pan.

4. Roast the onions and peppers in the preheated oven, stirring the onions twice, for 25 minutes, or until the onions caramelize and the peppers take on a black char.
5. Remove the vegetables from the oven and immediately place the peppers in a tightly sealed plastic bag for about 20 minutes to "sweat" them (loosen the skins). Let cool, then gently peel the skins off the peppers and slice into 1-inch-by-3-inch strips.
6. Grill the steaks over medium heat for about 5 minutes per side (for medium-rare meat). Tent the steaks in aluminum foil and let rest for 3 to 4 minutes.
7. Top the steaks with the roasted red peppers and onions, and serve.

Substitution tip: Other economical cuts of beef that work well in this recipe include strip steak, tri-tip, or even flank steak (though that has risen in price the past few years).

Pork Sirloin Roast with Mango-Apple Salsa

GLUTEN-FREE

SERVES 8

PREP TIME:
20 MINUTES

COOK TIME:
1 HOUR AND
40 MINUTES

Per serving
Calories: 195
Total Fat: 6g
Saturated Fat: <1g
Cholesterol: 30mg
Sodium: 10mg
Carbohydrates: 17g
Fiber: 2g
Protein: 23g

If you've never cooked or eaten a sirloin pork roast, you're in for a treat! This lean and tender cut of pork is versatile, and the salsa dresses it up for an elegant and interesting fruit-forward meal. Use the chilled salsa as a crisp and refreshing accent in the summer, or warm it up to create an incredible chutney in the cooler months.

FOR THE SALSA

2 (15-ounce) cans diced mangos in their own juice, drained (or 3 fresh mangos, diced)

½ cup diced apple

¼ cup diced red onion

¼ cup diced red bell pepper

2 teaspoons sugar

2 teaspoons white vinegar

¼ teaspoon red pepper flakes

FOR THE PORK

Cooking spray

2 tablespoons extra-virgin olive oil

2 teaspoons garlic powder

1 teaspoon dried thyme

½ teaspoon freshly ground black pepper

½ teaspoon Dijon mustard

2-pound pork sirloin tip roast

To make the salsa

In a medium bowl, combine the mangos, apple, red onion, bell pepper, sugar, vinegar, and red pepper flakes. Refrigerate while you cook the pork, or overnight.

To make the pork

1. Preheat the oven to 325°F. Line a sheet pan with aluminum foil and spray lightly with cooking spray.
2. In a small bowl, whisk together the olive oil, garlic powder, dried thyme, black pepper, and mustard.

3. Rub the outside of the pork with the olive oil mixture and place it on the foil-lined sheet pan. Roast the pork in the preheated oven for 1 hour and 40 minutes, or until just barely pink inside.

4. Remove from the oven and let rest a few minutes. Slice across the grain and serve with the salsa.

Leftover tip: Repurpose the leftovers of this roast to make sandwiches and use the salsa as a sandwich spread. You could also toss the leftover pork into a stir-fry with any veggies in your vegetable drawer or use it to make a quick soup or stew.

Broiled Sesame-Orange Beef

BUDGET-FRIENDLY

SERVES 8

PREP TIME:
15 MINUTES,
PLUS 24 TO
48 HOURS TO
MARINATE

COOK TIME:
15 MINUTES

Per serving
Calories: 199
Total Fat: 11g
Saturated Fat: 3g
Cholesterol: 34mg
Sodium: 31mg
Carbohydrates: 6g
Fiber: <1g
Protein: 20g

This flavor-filled marinade recipe is a great way to use lower-cost, less tender, lean cuts of beef but still enjoy the same robust flavor you would with more expensive cuts. Just plan ahead and marinate the beef for a day or two before you cook. Slicing this steak across the grain into thin strips and cooking it to medium-rare keeps it tender and juicy. Use any leftovers in sandwiches and salads.

⅓ cup diced red onion

¼ cup freshly squeezed orange juice

¼ cup frozen orange juice concentrate

2 tablespoons sesame oil

3 garlic cloves, chopped

1 tablespoon reduced-sodium soy sauce

1 teaspoon Dijon mustard

Zest of 1 orange

1½ pounds London broil steak (also called top round) or flank steak

1. In a small bowl, whisk together the onion, orange juice, orange juice concentrate, sesame oil, garlic, soy sauce, mustard, and orange zest.
2. Make ⅛-inch cuts in a large diamond pattern on each side of the steak to tenderize it and prepare it to absorb the marinade.
3. Put the steak in a nonreactive sealable container or a leakproof plastic bag and add the marinade. Seal the container and refrigerate. Marinate for 24 to 48 hours.
4. Place the oven rack 3 to 4 inches from the top heating element in the oven. Set the oven to broil. Drain the steak, put it on an aluminum foil–lined broiling pan or sheet pan, and broil for 10 to 12 minutes, turning once halfway through (for medium-rare meat).
5. Remove the steak from the oven, tent it with the foil, and let it rest for 5 minutes. Once rested, slice thinly across the grain before serving.

Rosemary-Orange Marinated Pork Tenderloin

SERVES 5

PREP TIME:
10 MINUTES,
PLUS 4 HOURS
TO OVERNIGHT
TO MARINATE

COOK TIME:
20 MINUTES

Per serving
Calories: 168
Total Fat: 10g
Saturated Fat: 2g
Cholesterol: 36mg
Sodium: 145mg
Carbohydrates: 4g
Fiber: <1g
Protein: 16g

You can grill this pork or simply roast it in the oven. Pork tenderloins often come in packages of two loins so be sure to double the marinade if you're cooking both (or if you buy a particularly large one). The flavor-filled marinade transforms into a serving sauce after heating, and you'll want every drop to drizzle on the tender pork.

½ cup orange juice

2 tablespoons extra-virgin olive oil

2 garlic cloves, chopped

1 tablespoon low-sodium soy sauce

1½ teaspoons dried rosemary

1 pound pork tenderloin

1. In a small bowl, whisk together the orange juice, olive oil, garlic, soy sauce, and rosemary to make the marinade.
2. Put the pork tenderloin in a nonreactive sealable container or a leakproof plastic bag and pour in the marinade. Marinate, refrigerated, for at least 4 hours, ideally overnight.
3. When ready to cook, drain the marinade into a small saucepan. Heat to boiling and boil for 3 minutes. (This kills any bacteria in the marinade so it can be reused as a sauce.) Reduce the heat and keep warm.
4. Grill the marinated pork tenderloin (or bake it in a preheated oven at 400°F) until the internal temperature reaches 145°F, 15 to 18 minutes. Serve with the warmed sauce.

Recipe tip: Use the delicious sauce to top mashed potatoes or any other starch you serve on the side.

Upside-Down Beef Cottage Pie

30 MINUTES | BUDGET-FRIENDLY | GLUTEN-FREE | TIME-SAVER

SERVES 5 TO 6

PREP TIME:
15 MINUTES

COOK TIME:
15 MINUTES

Per serving
Calories: 414
Total Fat: 12g
Saturated Fat: 5g
Cholesterol: 68mg
Sodium: 282mg
Carbohydrates: 50g
Fiber: 7g
Protein: 28g

You may have heard of shepherd's pie or cottage pie, a traditional English dish made with lamb and blanketed with a mashed potato topping. I've turned this recipe upside-down by using ground beef instead of lamb and putting the potatoes on the bottom instead of the top.

1 (24-ounce) bag baby red potatoes

½ cup light sour cream (or plain Greek yogurt)

1 cup low-sodium beef broth, plus 1 tablespoon

1½ teaspoons dry mustard, divided

2 teaspoons extra-virgin olive oil

1 pound lean ground beef

1 cup chopped onion

1½ cups frozen corn

1½ cups frozen peas

1½ cups frozen French-cut green beans

1½ cups frozen carrots

2 teaspoons garlic powder

¼ teaspoon freshly ground black pepper

4 tablespoons shredded light Cheddar cheese

1. Boil the potatoes as directed on the package, about 10 minutes, or until they're fork-tender and mashable.
2. Drain the potatoes and put them in a large bowl. Add the sour cream, 1 tablespoon of beef broth, and ½ teaspoon of dry mustard. Gently mash this mixture together, creating a rough mash. (Be careful not to create a gluey texture. Chunks are fine!) Set aside on the countertop.
3. Evenly brush the olive oil over the bottom and sides of a large pot or Dutch oven. Sauté the ground beef and onion over medium heat for 3 to 4 minutes, or until the onions are soft and the beef is browned.

4. Add the the remaining 1 cup of beef broth, the remaining 1 teaspoon of dry mustard, and the corn, peas, green beans, carrots, garlic, and black pepper. Cook for about 15 minutes, covered, stirring occasionally.

5. To serve, place a scoop of the mashed potatoes on a plate or in a bowl, and then spoon the beef-and-vegetable mixture over it. Sprinkle each serving with 1 tablespoon of Cheddar cheese.

Ingredient tip: Prewashed, precut frozen products deliver the same nutrients as fresh—sometimes even more! Take advantage of these amazing time- and energy-savers.

Stuffed Cauli-Peppers with Beef

GLUTEN-FREE

SERVES 4

PREP TIME:
10 MINUTES

COOK TIME:
30 MINUTES

Per serving
Calories: 308
Total Fat: 12g
Saturated Fat: 4g
Cholesterol: 74mg
Sodium: 234mg
Carbohydrates: 25g
Fiber: 8g
Protein: 29g

With this recipe, I've given the old favorite of rice-stuffed green bell peppers an upscale twist that lowers the carbs by using riced cauliflower (available in practically any frozen-foods aisle now). You won't even notice that the "rice" is cauliflower in disguise. It's a clever way to increase the vegetable power in your blood-pressure-lowering diet.

2 teaspoons extra-virgin olive oil

1 pound lean ground beef

½ cup chopped onion

3 garlic cloves, chopped

1 (10-ounce) bag frozen riced cauliflower

8 ounces tomato sauce (no salt added)

1 (6-ounce) can tomato paste (no salt added)

3 to 4 tablespoons water

1 teaspoon dried basil

1 teaspoon dried oregano

¼ teaspoon freshly ground black pepper

4 green bell peppers, seeded and cored

Cooking spray

4 tablespoons part-skim shredded mozzarella cheese, divided

1. Preheat the oven to 350°F.
2. Evenly brush a large skillet or sauté pan with the olive oil. Sauté the beef and onion over medium heat for about 5 minutes, or until the onion is soft and the beef is browned. Add the garlic and stir for 1 minute more.
3. Add the cauliflower rice, tomato sauce, tomato paste, water, basil, oregano, and black pepper. Stir to combine, adjusting the consistency with more water if needed. Cook for 2 to 3 minutes, then remove from the heat and set aside.
4. Stuff each pepper with one-quarter of the beef mixture, being sure to push the filling down all the way into the cavity of the pepper to completely fill it.

5. Spray an 8-inch glass baking pan with cooking spray. Place the peppers, spaced evenly, into the baking pan. Bake in the pre-heated oven, uncovered, for 15 minutes.

6. Sprinkle 1 tablespoon of the mozzarella cheese on top of each pepper and continue baking for 5 more minutes.

7. Let stand for 3 to 4 minutes before serving.

Substitution tip: This recipe can easily be made vegetarian by omitting the ground beef and substituting any type of low-sodium canned beans, drained and rinsed.

Beef and Vegetable Ragu over Polenta

BUDGET-FRIENDLY | GLUTEN-FREE | TIME-SAVER

SERVES 5 TO 6

PREP TIME:
15 MINUTES

COOK TIME:
35 MINUTES

Per serving
Calories: 351
Total Fat: 10g
Saturated Fat: 4g
Cholesterol: 61mg
Sodium: 266mg
Carbohydrates: 35g
Fiber: 6g
Protein: 24g

The deep comforting flavors of this hearty meal represent a variation on the classic Italian ragu sauce, but packed with nutrients for good health. With its lean ground beef and red wine, the tomato-y gravy is oh-so-yummy when it soaks into the polenta. Pairing it with artisan whole-wheat bread or pappardelle noodles instead of polenta is another great way to enjoy it.

2 teaspoons extra-virgin olive oil

1 pound lean ground beef

½ cup chopped onion

3 garlic cloves, chopped

½ cup grated carrots

½ cup chopped celery

1 (14.5-ounce) can low-sodium canned diced tomatoes

1 (8-ounce) can tomato sauce (no salt added)

1 (6-ounce) bag chopped frozen spinach

½ cup red wine

2 tablespoons tomato paste

1 tablespoon water

2 teaspoons Italian seasoning

4 servings polenta made from stone-ground cornmeal

¼ cup shredded Parmesan cheese

1. Evenly brush a large skillet with the olive oil. Sauté the ground beef and onion over medium heat for 3 to 4 minutes, until the beef is browned and the onion is soft.
2. Add the garlic and stir for about 1 minute, being careful not to let it brown.
3. Add the carrots and celery, followed by the diced tomatoes, tomato sauce, spinach, red wine, tomato paste, water, and Italian seasoning. Stir well. Cover and simmer on low for 30 minutes.

4. While the ragu simmers, cook 4 servings of polenta according to the package directions. (Don't add any salt or cheese.)
5. Just before serving, stir the Parmesan cheese into the ragu. Serve the ragu over the polenta in large bowls.

Ingredient tip: If you're short on time, buy ready-to-serve polenta in a tube (I like Bob's Red Mill), and simply slice and reheat it in a pan or the microwave.

Balsamic Beef-and-Vegetable Kebabs

BUDGET-FRIENDLY | GLUTEN-FREE

SERVES 8

PREP TIME:
15 MINUTES,
PLUS 4 HOURS
TO MARINATE

COOK TIME:
10 MINUTES

Per serving
Calories: 225
Total Fat: 15g
Saturated Fat: 4g
Cholesterol: 56mg
Sodium: 60mg
Carbohydrates: 6g
Fiber: 1g
Protein: 19g

These grilled kebabs are perfect for outdoor entertaining. The potent marinade renders the beef tender, and the balsamic vinegar gives both the meat and vegetables a pleasant tang. The four deliciously roasted veggies, along with a side salad, will keep your DASH veggie tally on track, too! I like serving these colorful skewers on a platter over brown or black rice.

FOR THE VEGETABLES

2 tablespoons extra-virgin olive oil

1 tablespoon balsamic vinegar

½ teaspoon dried basil

½ teaspoon dried oregano

⅛ teaspoon freshly ground black pepper

2 small zucchini

1 large red onion

12 small cherry tomatoes

12 small mushrooms

FOR THE BEEF

3 tablespoons extra-virgin olive oil

3 garlic cloves, minced

1 tablespoon balsamic vinegar

½ teaspoon Dijon mustard

½ teaspoon dried basil

½ teaspoon dried oregano

¼ teaspoon freshly ground black pepper

⅛ teaspoon red pepper flakes

1½ pounds beef tri-tip (strips), cut into 1½-inch pieces

2 tablespoons blue cheese (optional)

To make the vegetables

1. In a large bowl, whisk together the olive oil, vinegar, basil, oregano, and black pepper.
2. Cut the zucchini in half lengthwise, and then slice each half into 1-inch-wide half-moons.

3. Using a nonserrated knife, cut the peeled onion in half horizontally. Lay the halves cut-side down and quarter them. Cut each quarter in half one more time to make smaller, skewer-friendly pieces of onion.
4. Add the zucchini, onion, cherry tomatoes, and mushrooms to the bowl of marinade. Stir well and marinate, unrefrigerated, for 4 hours.

To make the beef
1. In a small bowl, whisk together the olive oil, garlic, vinegar, mustard, basil, oregano, black pepper, and red pepper flakes.
2. Put the pieces of beef in a nonreactive container or leakproof plastic bag with the marinade and marinate, refrigerated, for at least 4 hours.

To make the kebabs
1. Soak wooden skewers for at least 15 minutes in water before using (or use steel skewers). Alternate threading pieces of beef, onion, tomato, mushroom, and zucchini on the skewers. Repeat until all the beef and vegetables are skewered. Discard the leftover marinade.
2. Place the skewers on a grill over medium heat. For medium-rare meat, cook each side for 5 minutes. Cook longer for medium or well-done meat.
3. Place the skewers on a large platter. Sprinkle lightly with the blue cheese (if using) and serve.

Cooking tip: These kebabs may be cooked on a grill pan indoors as well.

New-Fashioned Meatloaf

BUDGET-FRIENDLY

SERVES 4

PREP TIME:
15 MINUTES

COOK TIME:
1 HOUR

Per serving
Calories: 279
Total Fat: 11g
Saturated Fat: 3g
Cholesterol: 117mg
Sodium: 126mg
Carbohydrates: 22g
Fiber: 3g
Protein: 26g

This is my mother's old-fashioned meatloaf recipe reinvented! I grew up with this charming Midwestern recipe—this meatloaf and a baked potato is still my favorite choice for a comfort food meal. Its texture and tomatoey goodness is hearty and satisfying down to the last bite. It's also freezer-friendly, so feel free to double the recipe!

1 pound lean ground beef (or ground turkey)

¾ cup old-fashioned oats

1 (8-ounce) can low-sodium tomato sauce, divided

1 large egg or 2 small eggs, beaten

½ cup chopped green bell pepper

¼ cup chopped yellow onion

1 teaspoon garlic powder

1 teaspoon dried basil

1 teaspoon dried oregano

⅛ teaspoon freshly ground black pepper

Cooking spray

2 tablespoons brown sugar

2 tablespoons white vinegar

1 teaspoon dry mustard (or 4 teaspoons yellow mustard)

½ cup water

1. Preheat the oven to 350°F.
2. In a large mixing bowl, with clean hands, gently combine the ground beef, oats, half the tomato sauce, egg, bell pepper, onion, garlic powder, basil, oregano, and black pepper. Be sure the ingredients are evenly distributed throughout the mixture. Don't overmix (the telltale sign of overmixing the ingredients is a "gummy" texture).
3. Spray a 9-inch loaf pan with cooking spray and put the meat mixture inside, shaping it to just fit the pan without pressing down hard. Use a fork to make a few holes in the meatloaf so it can absorb the sauce.

4. In a small bowl, whisk the remaining tomato sauce together with the brown sugar, vinegar, mustard, and water. Pour the sauce over the meat loaf.
5. Bake in the preheated oven for 1 hour. Remove and let stand for 5 minutes before serving.

Sweet-and-Sour Pork Stir-Fry

SERVES 4

PREP TIME:
10 MINUTES,
PLUS AT LEAST
20 MINUTES TO
MARINATE

COOK TIME:
10 MINUTES

Per serving
Calories: 316
Total Fat: 14g
Saturated Fat: 3g
Cholesterol: 53mg
Sodium: 219mg
Carbohydrates: 24g
Fiber: 4g
Protein: 21g

This recipe is healthier than the sweet-and-sour pork you get at restaurants because of the homemade stir-fry sauce—but that doesn't mean you'll sacrifice any flavor! It's bursting with fresh sweet pineapple and a plethora of crunchy vegetables that complement the tender and juicy pork. Every bite has a little heat and a little sweet!

FOR THE PORK

1 tablespoon dry sherry

1 tablespoon grated fresh ginger

1 teaspoon sesame oil

1 teaspoon low-sodium soy sauce

½ teaspoon sugar

⅛ teaspoon freshly ground black pepper

3 large thick-cut boneless pork loins

FOR THE STIR-FRY SAUCE

1 cup canned pineapple chunks in their own juice (no added sugar or syrup)

¼ cup water

2 tablespoons low-sodium tomato paste

¾ tablespoon sriracha sauce (use less for less heat)

1 teaspoon low-sodium soy sauce

1 teaspoon sesame oil

1 teaspoon sugar

⅛ teaspoon freshly ground black pepper

FOR THE STIR-FRY

4 teaspoons avocado (or peanut) oil, divided

2 cups snap peas

1 cup chopped celery

¾ cup mushrooms, sliced

1 red bell pepper, cut into narrow strips

½ cup chopped scallions

To make the pork

1. To make the marinade, in a small bowl, whisk together the sherry, ginger, sesame oil, soy sauce, sugar, and black pepper.
2. Slice the pork loins across the grain into ½-inch-thick slices. Put them in a large glass pan and pour the marinade over them. Marinate as long as possible, at least 20 minutes.

To make the stir-fry sauce

1. Strain the pineapple chunks, reserving the juice. Set the pineapple chunks aside.

2. In a medium bowl, whisk ¼ cup of the strained pineapple juice with the water, tomato paste, sriracha, soy sauce, sesame oil, sugar, and black pepper. Set aside.

To make the stir-fry

1. Evenly brush the bottom and sides of a wok or large skillet with 2 teaspoons of the avocado oil.

2. Heat the wok on medium-high heat until a drop of water explodes on the pan when tested. Gently pour the pork and liquid marinade into the pan, and stir-fry for 3 to 4 minutes, until all pieces of pork are browned. Remove the pork and set aside.

3. Add the remaining 2 teaspoons of avocado oil to the pan, followed by the snap peas, celery, mushrooms, bell pepper, and chopped scallions. Add the stir-fry sauce and pineapple chunks, and stir-fry on high heat for 3 to 4 minutes, stirring constantly.

4. Once the vegetables are tender-crisp (don't overcook!), add the pork back into the pan and mix everything together. Serve over brown rice, if desired.

Grilled Caribbean Flank Steak with Cilantro-Coconut Rice

BUDGET-FRIENDLY | GLUTEN-FREE | TIME-SAVER

SERVES 8

PREP TIME:
15 MINUTES,
PLUS AT LEAST
6 HOURS TO
MARINATE

COOK TIME:
10 MINUTES

Per serving
Calories: 371
Total Fat: 17g
Saturated Fat: 4g
Cholesterol: 34mg
Sodium: 78mg
Carbohydrates: 34g
Fiber: 2g
Protein: 22g

The bold flavors of the Caribbean in this marinated flank steak will take you to a faraway island and then back again for more. A distinctive spice blend comes through as potent but not as fiery-hot as jerk seasonings. Serve with cilantro-coconut rice and skewers of pineapple and watermelon chunks for a Caribbean feast!

½ cup pineapple juice (unsweetened)

¼ cup canola oil

3 tablespoons freshly squeezed lime juice

½ tablespoon brown sugar

1 teaspoon allspice

1 teaspoon paprika

1 teaspoon ground cumin

1 teaspoon garlic powder

1 teaspoon onion powder

⅛ to ¼ teaspoon cayenne pepper

1½ to 2 pounds flank steak

1 cup brown rice

2 cups light coconut milk

¼ cup chopped fresh cilantro

2 cups pineapple chunks (fresh or canned)

2 cups watermelon chunks

1. In a small bowl, whisk together the pineapple juice, canola oil, lime juice, brown sugar, allspice, paprika, cumin, garlic powder, onion powder, and cayenne to make the marinade.
2. Use a sharp knife to pierce holes in the flank steak on both sides to tenderize it and allow it to absorb the marinade. Put the steak in a nonreactive sealable container or a leakproof plastic bag with the marinade. Marinate for at least 6 hours (overnight for best results).
3. Cook the rice according to the package directions, but use the coconut milk instead of water. When the rice is cooked, add the cilantro and fluff before serving.

4. While the rice cooks, make fruit skewers. Thread the pineapple and watermelon chunks onto metal skewers. Grill them over medium heat for 2 minutes per side. Take them off the grill and set aside.
5. Grill the steak over medium heat, 5 minutes per side (for medium-rare meat).
6. Slice across the grain of the steak and serve over the rice, with the fruit skewers on the side.

Pork Loins with Velvety Whole-Grain Mustard Sauce

30 MINUTES

SERVES 4

PREP TIME:
10 MINUTES

COOK TIME:
15 MINUTES

Per serving
Calories: 313
Total Fat: 25g
Saturated Fat: 6g
Cholesterol: 56mg
Sodium: 415mg
Carbohydrates: 3g
Fiber: <1g
Protein: 23g

The velvety smooth, luxurious mustard sauce that accompanies these fork-tender pork loins requires little energy or time. I like to serve this dish with a chewy whole grain like farro, barley, or whole-grain rice pilaf to boost the fiber content.

3 teaspoons canola oil, divided

¼ cup chopped shallots

3 tablespoons extra-virgin olive oil

1 tablespoon balsamic vinegar

1 tablespoon whole-grain mustard

½ teaspoon ground sage

½ teaspoon dried oregano

¼ cup half-and-half

4 thick-cut boneless pork loins

Fresh parsley (optional)

1. Evenly brush a small sauté pan with 1 teaspoon of canola oil. Sauté the shallots on low heat for 3 to 4 minutes, until they're soft and clear but not brown. Add the olive oil, vinegar, mustard, sage, and oregano, and stir well over low heat.
2. Whisk in the half-and-half until the sauce becomes thickened and smooth. Remove from the heat.

3. Evenly brush a large sauté pan with the remaining 2 teaspoons of canola oil. Cook the pork over medium heat for 4 minutes per side, or until the internal temperature reaches 145°F.
4. When the pork is done, tent the loins in aluminum foil and let rest for 3 minutes. Serve each individual pork loin topped with the savory mustard sauce and sprinkled with fresh parsley (if using).

Cooking tip: Pork can be served pink with no fear of causing foodborne illness, so don't overcook. Lean pork will stay juicy, tender, and flavorful when cooked properly to an internal temperature of 145°F followed by a 3-minute rest time.

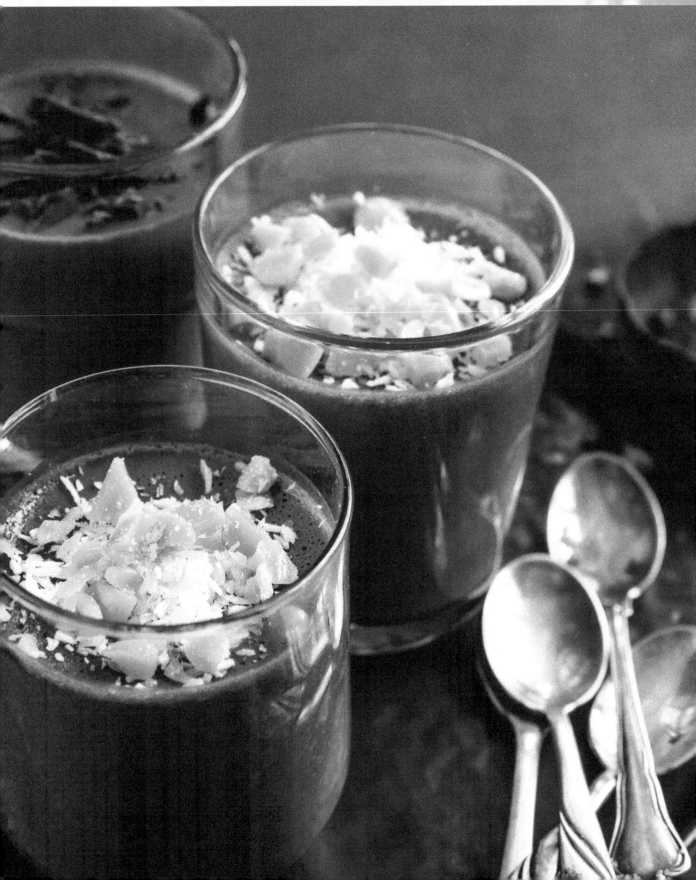

chapter nine

SNACKS AND SWEETS

◀ Chocolate-Coconut
Pots de Crème, *page 150*

Four-Ingredient Homemade Trail Mix

1 POT | 30 MINUTES | BUDGET-FRIENDLY | GLUTEN-FREE TIME-SAVER | VEGETARIAN

MAKES 2 CUPS

PREP TIME:
5 MINUTES

Per ½ cup serving
Calories: 280
Total Fat: 14g
Saturated Fat: 1g
Cholesterol: 0mg
Sodium: 65mg
Carbohydrates: 33g
Fiber: 7g
Protein: 7g

One of the healthiest and quickest snacks you can make at home is trail mix. You can mix and match any flavors you want—you just need a whole grain, an unsalted nut, an unsalted seed, and a dried fruit with no sugar or salt added. Eat this trail mix as is (delicious!) or with low-fat Greek yogurt or milk (amazing!). The nuts add antioxidants and healthy fats to reduce your risk of heart disease.

1 cup Nature's Path Honey Almond Granola

½ cup unsalted sliced almonds (or any unsalted nut)

¼ cup low-sugar dried cranberries (or any dried fruit with no sugar or salt added)

¼ cup unsalted sunflower seeds (or any unsalted seeds)

Combine the granola, almonds, cranberries, and sunflower seeds in a bowl or airtight bag. Shake or stir to mix. Store your trail mix in an airtight container to retain freshness.

Ingredient tip: Many whole-grain cereals are high in salt, but Nature's Path makes a line of low-sodium cereals containing a variety of whole grains, nuts, and seeds.

Spinach and Chickpea Dip

**30 MINUTES | BUDGET-FRIENDLY | GLUTEN-FREE
TIME-SAVER | VEGAN**

**MAKES
1½ CUPS**

PREP TIME:
10 MINUTES

**Per
2 tablespoons
serving**
Calories: 66
Total Fat: 3g
Saturated Fat: <1g
Cholesterol: 0mg
Sodium: 12mg
Carbohydrates: 8g
Fiber: 2g
Protein: 3g

This is an appetizing, health-forward alternative to high-calorie dips and spreads, and is great with raw vegetables or whole-wheat pita chips or bread. Having something tasty in which to dip your veggies helps motivate you to up your vegetable intake, which helps reduce your blood pressure and may even lower your weight.

1 (14.5-ounce) can low-sodium chickpeas, drained

6 ounces frozen flat-leaf spinach

2 tablespoons extra-virgin olive oil

2 tablespoons freshly squeezed lemon juice

1 tablespoon white balsamic vinegar

2 small garlic cloves, finely chopped

1 tablespoon water

¼ teaspoon freshly ground black pepper

1. Strain the chickpeas, reserving ¼ cup of the juice (called aquafaba).
2. In a blender, combine the reserved aquafaba with the chickpeas, spinach, olive oil, lemon juice, vinegar, garlic, water, and black pepper. Blend until very smooth. (It may take a few tries to get the frozen spinach to blend thoroughly into the other ingredients.)
3. Serve with your favorite raw veggies, whole-wheat pita chips, or homemade tortilla chips (see page 90).

Cottage Cheese, Chive, and Tomato Salad

30 MINUTES | BUDGET-FRIENDLY | VEGETARIAN

SERVES 4

PREP TIME:
5 MINUTES

Per serving
Calories: 65
Total Fat: 1g
Saturated Fat: 1g
Cholesterol: 15mg
Sodium: 339mg
Carbohydrates: 5g
Fiber: <1g
Protein: 10g

If you're a cottage cheese lover like I am, here's another way to get your craving met. This is a high-protein, blood-pressure-lowering snack that's filling enough to help you avoid mindless munching. It's also an easy way to increase your dairy intake to meet DASH diet guidelines.

1½ cups low-fat cottage cheese

½ cup halved cherry tomatoes

2 tablespoons chopped fresh chives (or scallion)

¼ teaspoon freshly ground black pepper

In a medium bowl, combine the cottage cheese, cherry tomatoes, chives, and pepper. Divide into four bowls and serve.

Substitution tip: Cottage cheese can easily go from savory to sweet. Try leaving out the black pepper and swapping out the veggies for fresh or canned fruit (in its own juice, no sugar added) to up your fruit intake.

Spiced Honey-Roasted Pecans

30 MINUTES | GLUTEN-FREE | VEGAN

MAKES 3 CUPS

PREP TIME:
3 MINUTES

COOK TIME:
10 MINUTES

**Per ¼ cup
serving**
Calories: 200
Total Fat: 21g
Saturated Fat: 2g
Cholesterol: 0mg
Sodium: 17mg
Carbohydrates: 5g
Fiber: 3g
Protein: 3g

These fast-to-fix pecans will be a hit at every party. They're also delicious chopped and sprinkled into salads. Their amazing flavor may astonish you, because there's no salt in them whatsoever! Plus they contain healthy fats, protein, antioxidants, and fiber that all come together to lower your risk of many diseases, including high blood pressure. Wouldn't they make a great housewarming or holiday gift?

3 cups unsalted raw pecan halves

1 tablespoon extra-virgin olive oil

1 teaspoon Frank's RedHot Original Cayenne Pepper Sauce

1 teaspoon Mrs. Dash Garlic and Herb seasoning

1 teaspoon Jane's Krazy Mixed-Up Pepper

1 teaspoon freshly ground black pepper

1½ teaspoons honey

1. Preheat the oven to 350°F.
2. While the oven is preheating, in a medium bowl, combine the pecans and olive oil, and stir well. Add the hot sauce and stir well. Then add the Mrs. Dash Garlic and Herb seasoning, the Jane's Krazy Mixed-Up Pepper seasoning, and the black pepper. Toss to coat.
3. Spread the spiced pecans out on a large baking pan. Drizzle the honey equally over all the pecans.
4. Place the pan on the center rack of the preheated oven and bake for 5 minutes. Then stir the pecans and bake for another 5 minutes, watching carefully to make sure they don't burn.
5. Remove the pecans from the oven and give them one last stir. Let cool before serving.

Chocolate-Coconut Pots de Crème

BUDGET-FRIENDLY | GLUTEN-FREE | VEGAN

SERVES 6

PREP TIME:
10 MINUTES,
PLUS 4 HOURS
TO CHILL

COOK TIME:
5 MINUTES

Per serving
Calories: 367
Total Fat: 23g
Saturated Fat: 15g
Cholesterol: 32mg
Sodium: 55mg
Carbohydrates: 40g
Fiber: <1g
Protein: 2g

Who says you can't enjoy a fancy chocolate dessert just because you have high blood pressure? These easy but elegant pots de crème have a deep chocolate flavor accentuated by unsweetened shredded coconut and the super sweet crunch of the toffee bits. I serve these a lot—they're perfect for dinner parties.

1 egg

1 teaspoon vanilla extract

1 (13.5-ounce) can light coconut milk

1½ cups semisweet chocolate chips, divided

1½ tablespoons toffee bits

6 teaspoons unsweetened shredded dried coconut

1. In a small bowl, beat the egg with the vanilla extract. Set aside.
2. Shake the coconut milk, then pour it into a small saucepan on the stove. Heat the milk to a rolling boil over medium-high heat. Boil, stirring constantly, for 3 to 4 minutes.
3. In a blender, put half of the chocolate chips. IMPORTANT: Remove the center piece of the lid of your blender to allow the steam to escape and prevent an explosion when you add the hot liquid.
4. Pour half of the hot milk into the blender over the chips, and then cover tightly with the vented lid. Place a dry towel on top of the lid and hold it down with your hand. Start the blender on the lowest setting for 15 seconds, then at an increased speed for another 15 seconds.
5. Next, add the egg and vanilla mixture, the remaining chips, and the rest of the milk, covering again with the vented lid and towel. Blend again, starting on the lowest setting first (about 15 seconds) then increase the speed for another 15 seconds.

6. Pour the chocolate mixture into 6 small ramekins and refrigerate for at least 4 hours, or ideally overnight, to set.

7. Before serving, sprinkle toffee bits and shredded coconut on top of each pot.

Preparation tip: Your blender must be made of glass and able to tolerate scalding liquids so that it doesn't crack or become damaged when you make this recipe. You can always opt for a hand blender instead.

Grilled Pineapple with Maple-Pecan Drizzle

**1 POT | 30 MINUTES | BUDGET-FRIENDLY | GLUTEN-FREE
TIME-SAVER | VEGAN**

SERVES 4

PREP TIME:
5 MINUTES

COOK TIME:
10 MINUTES

Per serving
Calories: 84
Total Fat: 4g
Saturated Fat: 1g
Cholesterol: 0mg
Sodium: 6mg
Carbohydrates: 13g
Fiber: 1g
Protein: <1g

A small drizzle of maple syrup adds a bit of extra sweetness to the natural sugars of grilled pineapple to create a heavenly finish to your meal. The toasted pecans are the perfect crunchy topper for this amazingly simple dessert.

**1 (8-ounce) can pineapple slices
(in their own juice, no sugar
added), drained**

**2 teaspoons extra-virgin
olive oil, divided**

4 teaspoons maple syrup, divided

**4 teaspoons unsalted toasted
pecans, divided**

1. Pat each slice of pineapple dry and evenly brush each side of the pineapple slice with olive oil, using a total of ½ teaspoon of olive oil per slice.
2. On a grill pan, over medium heat, grill the pineapple for 5 minutes on each side.
3. Remove from the heat and drizzle each pineapple slice with ½ teaspoon of syrup. Top each slice with ½ teaspoon of pecans.

Cooking tip: If you don't have a grill pan, a griddle does the trick, although you won't get the beautiful grill marks. You can also put them on an outdoor grill, if you have one.

Strawberries with Honey-Cream Topping

1 POT | BUDGET-FRIENDLY | GLUTEN-FREE | VEGETARIAN

SERVES 4

PREP TIME:
5 MINUTES,
PLUS
30 MINUTES
TO FREEZE

Per serving
Calories: 108
Total Fat: 3g
Saturated Fat: 2g
Cholesterol: 10mg
Sodium: 7mg
Carbohydrates: 19g
Fiber: 2g
Protein: 3g

It's easy to make fruit your dessert of choice when you dress it up and make it special. This fluffy and light whipped topping does just that and is great on any fruit—not just strawberries. The secret is the evaporated milk, which creates delicate cloud-like peaks of whipped cream. Any fresh or frozen fruit will add important nutrients to your diet, so take advantage of using this healthier topper to eat more fruit—with no guilt!

½ cup evaporated milk (unsweetened)

2 tablespoons light sour cream

1 teaspoon honey

½ teaspoon vanilla extract

2 cups fresh strawberries

1. Pour the evaporated milk into a medium glass bowl and put it in the freezer with the beaters you'll use to whip the topping. Freeze for 30 minutes.
2. Remove and beat with a hand mixer or immersion blender until soft peaks form. Add the sour cream, honey, and vanilla, and beat again, briefly, to combine. (This won't be a typical stiff whipped-cream texture, but very soft, more like a topping.)
3. Divide the strawberries into 4 serving dishes, cover each serving with a big dollop of topping, and serve.

Ingredient tip: Using evaporated milk instead of heavy cream in this recipe saves 75 calories and 7 grams of saturated fat per serving. It's also low in sodium and provides the same nutrients as milk.

Peach-Blueberry Oatmeal Crumble

BUDGET-FRIENDLY | TIME-SAVER | VEGETARIAN

SERVES 4 TO 6

PREP TIME:
10 MINUTES

COOK TIME:
45 MINUTES

Per serving
Calories: 235
Total Fat: 13g
Saturated Fat: 7g
Cholesterol: 31mg
Sodium: 75mg
Carbohydrates: 31g
Fiber: 3g
Protein: 3g

I love using fruit for desserts because it adds to the healthful tally of 10 servings of fruits and veggies a day recommended by the DASH diet. Yes, this recipe is a splurge because of the unsalted butter and ¼ teaspoon of salt, but that's what a dessert is—a splurge and not something you eat every day or every week.

Cooking spray

2 cups frozen sliced peaches (no sugar or syrup)

2 cups frozen blueberries (no sugar or syrup)

¾ cup old-fashioned oats

½ cup flour

½ cup sugar

¾ teaspoon ground cinnamon

¼ teaspoon kosher salt

4 ounces unsalted butter, at room temperature

1. Preheat the oven to 350°F.
2. Spray an 8-inch-by-8-inch glass baking pan with the cooking spray.
3. In a small bowl, stir the peaches and blueberries together, then pour into the baking pan (while still frozen).
4. In a large bowl, mix together the oats, flour, sugar, cinnamon, and salt. Cut the butter into this mixture and combine until it's crumbly.

5. Sprinkle the oat mixture evenly onto the top of the fruit mixture and bake in the preheated oven for 45 minutes. Remove and let sit for 5 minutes to allow the fruit juices to set. Distribute among 4 bowls, and serve on its own or with a small scoop of low-fat vanilla ice cream.

Ingredient tip: Frozen fruit has as many nutrients as fresh (or more), so don't be afraid to use it to help reach your daily fruit goals on the DASH diet.

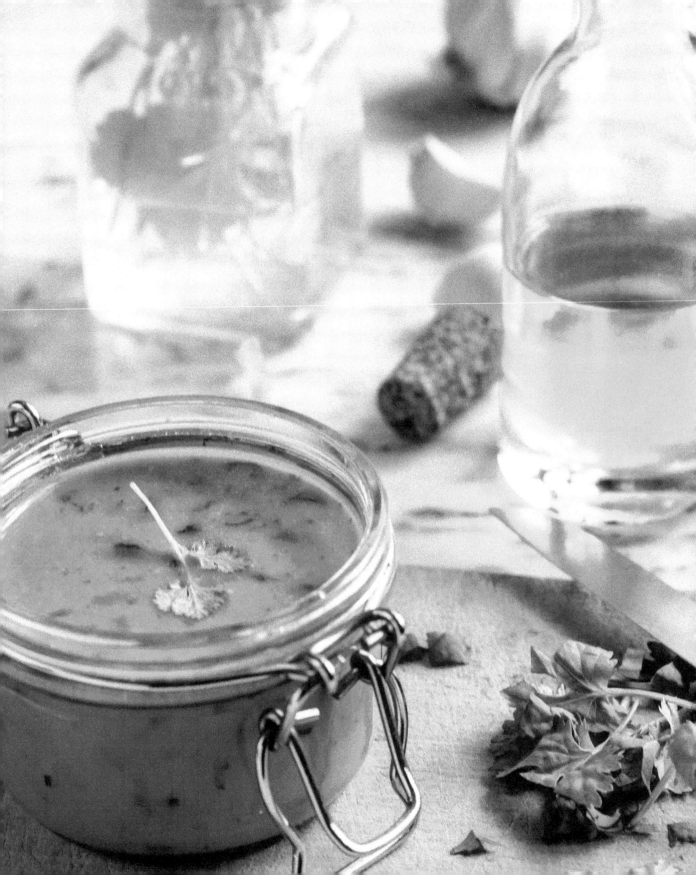

chapter ten

SAUCES AND DRESSINGS

30-Minute Marinara

1 POT | 30 MINUTES | BUDGET-FRIENDLY | VEGAN

MAKES 5 CUPS

PREP TIME:
5 MINUTES

COOK TIME:
25 MINUTES

Per serving
(½ cup)
Calories: 96
Total Fat: 5g
Saturated Fat: 1g
Cholesterol: <1mg
Sodium: 67mg
Carbohydrates: 11g
Fiber: <1g
Protein: 2g

Tomatoes contain lycopene, which has been shown in clinical studies to lower systolic blood pressure by 5 mmHg (when intake is at least 25 milligrams per day) and to reduce the risk of stroke by 59 percent. Eating tomatoes with olive oil greatly increases your body's ability to absorb it. This sauce is not only delicious and healthy—it's freezer-friendly, too!

3½ tablespoons extra-virgin olive oil, divided

1 cup chopped yellow onion

4 garlic cloves, chopped

1 (29-ounce) can low-sodium tomato purée (or tomato purée with no salt in the ingredients)

1 cup water

2 tablespoons tomato paste

1 tablespoon dried basil

1 tablespoon dried oregano

½ tablespoon dried thyme

½ teaspoon sugar

½ teaspoon balsamic vinegar

¼ teaspoon freshly ground black pepper

1 tablespoon shredded Parmesan cheese

1. Evenly brush the bottom and sides of a sauté pan with 2 tablespoons of the olive oil. Over low heat, sauté the onion until it's clear and soft, about 3 minutes. Add the chopped garlic and sauté, stirring frequently, for 1 minute.
2. Add 1 tablespoon of olive oil, tomato purée, water, tomato paste, basil, oregano, thyme, sugar, vinegar, and black pepper.
3. Simmer for about 20 minutes, until thickened. Just before serving, stir in the Parmesan cheese and remaining ½ tablespoon of olive oil.

Onion and Herb Buttermilk Salad Dressing

30 MINUTES | BUDGET-FRIENDLY | GLUTEN-FREE | VEGETARIAN

MAKES 1 CUP

PREP TIME:
10 MINUTES

Per serving
(1 tablespoon)
Calories: 25
Total Fat: 2g
Saturated Fat: <1g
Cholesterol: <1mg
Sodium: 21mg
Carbohydrates: 1g
Fiber: 0g
Protein: <1g

This dressing is creamy, but not heavy, with a mellow but tangy taste that superbly coats every green leaf in your salad. I especially like it on spring greens with radishes, tomatoes, and cucumbers because it pumps up the vegetable flavors. You can also drizzle it on cooked veggies, pasta, or poached fish.

¾ cup buttermilk

2 tablespoons extra-virgin olive oil

1½ tablespoons light mayonnaise

1 tablespoon chopped fresh scallion

2 teaspoons freshly squeezed lemon juice

1½ teaspoons onion powder

1 teaspoon sugar

½ teaspoon freshly ground black pepper

½ teaspoon fresh oregano

1 to 2 teaspoons chopped fresh chives

1. In a blender, blend the buttermilk, olive oil, mayonnaise, scallion, lemon juice, onion powder, sugar, black pepper, and oregano for 1 minute.
2. Stir in the chives and chill before serving to allow the flavors to meld.

Storage tip: This dressing gets even better and brighter as it sits in your refrigerator. Just shake or stir before using.

Easy Honey-Dijon Sauce

1 POT | 30 MINUTES | BUDGET-FRIENDLY | VEGETARIAN

MAKES ½ CUP

PREP TIME:
5 MINUTES

Per serving
(2 tablespoons)
Calories: 103
Total Fat: 7g
Saturated Fat: 1g
Cholesterol: 0mg
Sodium: 184mg
Carbohydrates: 10g
Fiber: 0g
Protein: 0g

This lively and versatile honey-mustard sauce is delicious on just about anything! It livens up fish, chicken, or any cooked or roasted vegetable, and can also be used as a simple salad dressing.

4 tablespoons freshly squeezed lemon juice

2 tablespoons honey

2 tablespoons Dijon mustard

2 tablespoons extra-virgin olive oil

In a small bowl, whisk together the lemon juice, honey, mustard, and olive oil until fully combined.

Lemon-Garlic Vinaigrette

1 POT | 30 MINUTES | VEGAN

MAKES 1 CUP

PREP TIME:
5 MINUTES

Per serving
(1 tablespoon)
Calories: 64
Total Fat: 7g
Saturated Fat: 1g
Cholesterol: 0mg
Sodium: <1mg
Carbohydrates: 1g
Fiber: 0g
Protein: 0g

This simple dressing enhances everything it touches, from grains to greens to pasta salads. Chances are you already have all the ingredients in your refrigerator or pantry and can pull this together in 5 minutes. No worries if you don't have a shallot on hand—you can use any other onion you already have.

½ cup freshly squeezed lemon juice

½ cup extra-virgin olive oil

½ tablespoon maple syrup

1 teaspoon chopped fresh garlic

½ teaspoon freshly ground black pepper

1 small shallot, chopped

1. In a blender, blend the lemon juice, olive oil, maple syrup, garlic, and pepper for 1 minute until smooth.
2. Add the chopped shallot and stir. Pour into a container and chill before serving.

Chipotle-Orange Sauce with Cilantro

30 MINUTES | BUDGET-FRIENDLY | TIME-SAVER | VEGAN

MAKES 2 CUPS

PREP TIME:
10 MINUTES

COOK TIME:
5 MINUTES

Per serving
(2 tablespoons)
Calories: 47
Total Fat: 2g
Saturated Fat: <1g
Cholesterol: 0mg
Sodium: 20mg
Carbohydrates: 7g
Fiber: 0g
Protein: 0g

The intense orange flavor combined with the smoky kick of the chipotle in this recipe is a winning combination if you like a little sweet heat. This sauce complements scallops, shrimp, white fish, chicken, and tofu—not to mention raw or steamed vegetables.

6 ounces orange juice concentrate (undiluted)

¼ cup orange juice

2 tablespoons maple syrup

2 tablespoons extra-virgin olive oil

1 tablespoon chipotle pepper with adobo sauce (from a can)

1 tablespoon yellow mustard

1 teaspoon chopped garlic

2 teaspoons chopped fresh cilantro (optional)

1. In a blender, blend the orange juice concentrate, orange juice, maple syrup, olive oil, chipotle, mustard, and garlic for 1 minute.
2. Stir in the chopped cilantro (if using).
3. Transfer the sauce to a small saucepan and gently heat on low until warm, 2 to 3 minutes.

Substitution tip: For a less spicy sauce, use only ½ teaspoon of chipotle and drain it first. If you don't like cilantro, try fresh oregano or basil instead.

Everyday Herb Vinaigrette

30 MINUTES | GLUTEN-FREE | VEGETARIAN

**MAKES
2½ CUPS**

PREP TIME:
5 TO 10
MINUTES, PLUS
1 TO 2 HOURS
TO CHILL

Per serving
(1 tablespoon)
Calories: 45
Total Fat: 5g
Saturated Fat: <1g
Cholesterol: 0mg
Sodium: 10mg
Carbohydrates: 1g
Fiber: 0g
Protein: 0g

A friend gave me the original recipe for this salad dressing, and I've enjoyed tweaking it a bit to bump up the taste. It's a wonderfully smooth, herbaceous, balanced vinaigrette that will enhance any salad. It has become one of my favorite salad dressings and I hope it becomes one of yours!

¾ cup extra-virgin olive oil

⅓ cup white balsamic vinegar

2 garlic cloves, finely chopped

1 tablespoon Dijon mustard

1 tablespoon honey

½ teaspoon dried basil

½ teaspoon dried oregano

¼ teaspoon freshly ground black pepper

Pinch cayenne pepper

1. In a medium bowl, whisk together the olive oil, vinegar, garlic, mustard, honey, basil, oregano, black pepper, and cayenne pepper.
2. Pour into a glass jar with a tight lid and refrigerate for 1 to 2 hours to blend the flavors. Before using, let warm on the counter for 30 minutes and shake before use. Store in the refrigerator for up to 2 weeks.

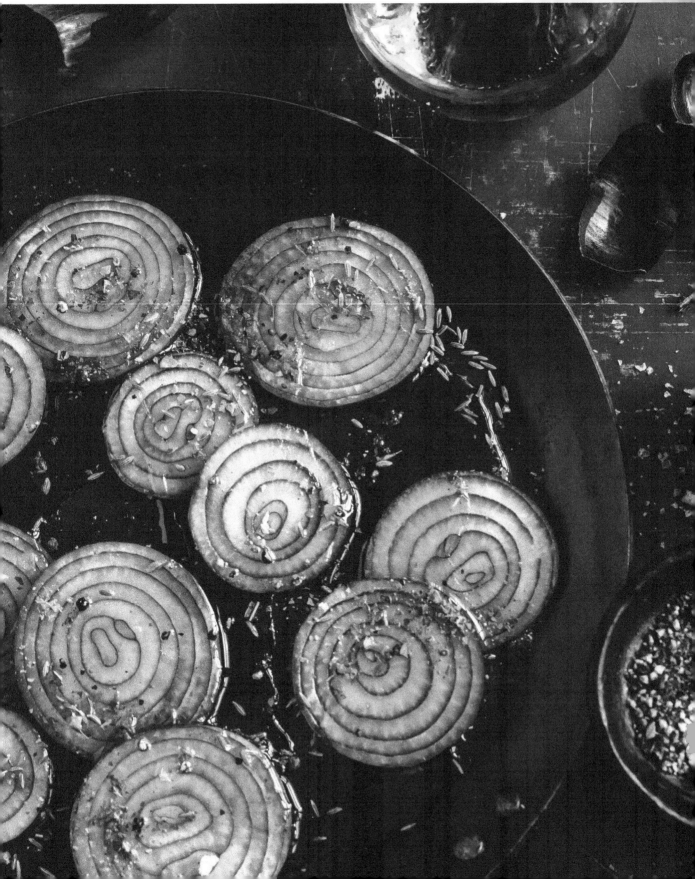

MEASUREMENT CONVERSIONS

VOLUME EQUIVALENTS (LIQUID)

US STANDARD	US STANDARD (OUNCES)	METRIC (APPROX.)
2 tablespoons	1 fl. oz.	30 mL
¼ cup	2 fl. oz.	60 mL
½ cup	4 fl. oz.	120 mL
1 cup	8 fl. oz.	240 mL
1½ cups	12 fl. oz.	355 mL
2 cups or 1 pint	16 fl. oz.	475 mL
4 cups or 1 quart	32 fl. oz.	1 L
1 gallon	128 fl. oz.	4 L

OVEN TEMPERATURES

FAHRENHEIT (F)	CELSIUS (C) (APPROX.)
250°F	120°C
300°F	150°C
325°F	165°C
350°F	180°C
375°F	190°C
400°F	200°C
425°F	220°C
450°F	230°C

VOLUME EQUIVALENTS (DRY)

US STANDARD	METRIC (APPROX.)
⅛ teaspoon	0.5 mL
¼ teaspoon	1 mL
½ teaspoon	2 mL
¾ teaspoon	4 mL
1 teaspoon	5 mL
1 tablespoon	15 mL
¼ cup	59 mL
⅓ cup	79 mL
½ cup	118 mL
⅔ cup	156 mL
¾ cup	177 mL
1 cup	235 mL
2 cups or 1 pint	475 mL
3 cups	700 mL
4 cups or 1 quart	1 L

WEIGHT EQUIVALENTS

US STANDARD (OUNCES)	METRIC (APPROX.)
½ ounce	15 g
1 ounce	30 g
2 ounces	60 g
4 ounces	115 g
8 ounces	225 g
12 ounces	340 g
16 ounces or 1 pound	455 g

RESOURCES

The Academy of Nutrition and Dietetics

www.eatright.org

Learn about nutrition and find a registered dietitian nutritionist (RDN) near you

The American Heart Association

www.heart.org

Info on managing blood pressure with a heart-healthy diet

The Centers for Disease Control and Prevention

www.cdc.gov/bloodpressure/index.htm

A wealth of information on high blood pressure

Choose My Plate

www.choosemyplate.org

USDA guidelines on food groups, portion sizes, and more, including for those with high blood pressure

The Healthy Heart Market

healthyheartmarket.com

More than 500 low-sodium products are available, including seasonings, baking products, condiments, sauces, staples, and more

The Mayo Clinic's DASH Diet Sample Menu

www.mayoclinic.org/healthy-lifestyle/nutrition-and-healthy-eating/in-depth /dash-diet/art-20047110

More ideas for blood pressure–friendly meals and snacks

REFERENCES

American College of Cardiology. "Know Your Numbers." Cardiosmart.org. Accessed August 28, 2019. https://www.cardiosmart.org/Healthy-Living /Know-your-Numbers.

American Heart Association. "American Heart Association Recommendations for Physical Activity in Adults and Kids." Accessed September 5, 2019. https: //www.heart.org/en/healthy-living/fitness/fitness-basics/aha-recs-for-physical-activity-in-adults.

American Heart Association. "Answers by Heart Fact Sheets." Accessed August 28, 2019. https://www.heart.org/en/health-topics/consumer-healthcare /answers-by-heart-fact-sheets.

American Heart Association. "2017 Hypertension Clinical Guidelines." Accessed August 28, 2019. https://professional.heart.org/professional/Science-News/UCM_496965_2017-Hypertension-Clinical-Guidelines.jsp.

American Heart Association. "Hypertension Guideline Resources." Last updated October 26, 2018. https://www.heart.org/en/health-topics/high-blood-pressure /high-blood-pressure-toolkit-resources.

Centers for Disease Control and Prevention. "2017 Hypertension Clinical Practice Guidelines Released." Accessed August 28, 2019. https://www.cdc.gov /bloodpressure/2017-htn-guidelines.htm.

Centers for Disease Control and Prevention, Division for Heart Disease and Stroke Prevention. "High Blood Pressure Fact Sheet." Last updated June 16, 2016. https://www.cdc.gov/dhdsp/data_statistics/fact_sheets/fs_bloodpres-sure.htm.

Charles, Lesley, Jean Triscott, and Bonnie Dobbs. "Secondary Hypertension: Discovering the Underlying Cause." *American Family Physician* 96, no. 7 (October 2017): 453–461. https://www.aafp.org/afp/2017/1001/p453.html.

Cheng, Ho Ming, Georgios Koutsidis, John K. Lodge, Ammar Ashor, Mario Siervo, and José Lara. "Tomato and Lycopene Supplementation and Cardiovascular Risk Factors: A Systematic Review and Meta-Analysis." *Atherosclerosis* 257 (February 2017): 100–108. https://doi.org/10.1016/j.atherosclerosis.2017.01.009.

Harvard Medical School. "Reading the New Blood Pressure Guidelines." Harvard Health Publishing. Accessed August 28, 2019. https://www.health.harvard.edu/heart-health/reading-the-new-blood-pressure-guidelines.

Harvard Medical School. "Should I Take a Potassium Supplement?" Harvard Health Publishing. Last updated June 24, 2019. https://www.health.harvard.edu/staying-healthy/should-i-take-a-potassium-supplement.

Johns Hopkins Medicine. "Combination Low-Salt and Heart-Healthy 'Dash' Diet as Effective as Drugs for Some Adults with High Blood Pressure." November 22, 2017. https://www.hopkinsmedicine.org/news/media/releases/combination_low_salt_and_heart_healthy_dash_diet_as_effective_as_drugs_for_some_adults_with_high_blood_pressure.

The Mayo Clinic. "High Blood Pressure (Hypertension)." Accessed August 28, 2019. https://www.mayoclinic.org/diseases-conditions/high-blood-pressure/diagnosis-treatment/drc-20373417.

National Institutes of Health, National Heart, Lung, and Blood Institute. "DASH Eating Plan." Accessed August 28, 2019. https://www.nhlbi.nih.gov/health-topics/dash-eating-plan.

National Institutes of Health, National Heart, Lung, and Blood Institute. *Your Guide to Lowering Your Blood Pressure with DASH.* NIH Publication no. 06–4082. Revised April 2006. https://www.nhlbi.nih.gov/files/docs/public/heart/new_dash.pdf.

National Kidney Foundation. "What Is High Blood Pressure?" Accessed August 28, 2019. https://www.kidney.org/atoz/what-high-blood-pressure.

Preventive Cardiovascular Nurses Association. "Blood Pressure: How Do You Measure Up?" Accessed August 28, 2019. https://pcna.net/clinical-resources /patient-handouts/hypertension-patient-tools-and-handouts.

Rodriguez-Mateos, A., C. Rendeiro, T. Bergillos-Meca, S. Tabatabaee, T. W. George, C. Heiss, and J. P. Spencer. "Intake and Time Dependence of Blueberry Flavonoid-Induced Improvements in Vascular Function: A Randomized, Controlled, Double-Blind, Crossover Intervention Study with Mechanistic Insights into Biological Activity." *The American Journal of Clinical Nutrition* 98, no. 5 (September 2013): 1179–91. doi: 10.3945/ajcn.113.066639.

Rodriguez-Mateos A, G. Istas, L. Boshchek, R. P. Feliciano, C. E. Mills, C. Boby, S. Gome-Alonso, D. Milenkovic, and C. Heiss. "Circulating Anthocyanin Metabolites Mediate Vascular Benefits of Blueberries: Insights from Randomized Controlled Trials, Metabolomics, and Nutrigenomics." *The Journals of Gerontology: Series A, Biological Sciences and Medical Sciences* 74, no. 7 (June 2019): 967–976. doi:10.1093/gerona/glz047.

United States Department of Agriculture, Agricultural Research Service. *USDA Food Composition Databases.* Accessed August 28, 2019. https://ndb.nal.usda .gov/ndb/.

Viera, Anthony J., and Dana M. Neutze. "Diagnosis of Secondary Hypertension: An Age-based Approach. American Academy of Family Physicians." *American Family Physician* 82, no. 12 (December 2010): 1471–1478. https://www.aafp.org /afp/2010/1215/p1471.html.

Whelton, PK, R. M. Carey, W. S. Aronow, D. E. Casey Jr, K, J. Collins, C. Dennison Himmelfarb, S. M. DePalma, et al. "2017 ACC/AHA/AAPA/ABC/ACPM /AGS/APhA/ASH/ASPC/NMA/PCNA guideline for the prevention, detection, evaluation, and management of high blood pressure in adults: a report of the American College of Cardiology/American Heart Association Task Force on Clinical Practice Guidelines." J Am Coll Cardiol 2018;71:e127–248.

INDEX

ACKNOWLEDGMENTS

I'd like to thank my husband for his good-natured sampling of the recipes in this book, and I'd also like to thank three special women in my "culinary sisterhood" who continually inspire and delight me with their amazing culinary skills. Thank you, Miriam Molver, for your gourmet cooking, which I've admired and enjoyed for the last 25 years! I truly appreciate your friendship and the gentle and thoughtful feedback you gave me on many of the recipes I developed for this book. And thank you to my sister-in-law, Cathy Nelson, and my other sister at heart, Karen Walker, for your support, encouragement, and cheerleading as I wrote this book.

ABOUT THE AUTHOR

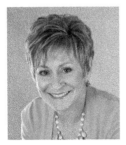

Kim Larson, RDN, NBC-HWC, is a registered dietitian nutritionist and board-certified health and wellness coach in the Seattle, Washington, area. Her company, Total Health, provides personalized health and lifestyle coaching for women, as well as public speaking, media spokesperson, and consulting services. Kim's areas of expertise include sports nutrition, weight management for men and women, and medical nutrition therapy for health conditions such as heart disease, high cholesterol, and high blood pressure. She writes a monthly column for the *Everett Herald* and is featured as a weekly guest on Health Beat, a KOMO News-Radio program in Seattle. You can find her online at www.totalhealthrd.com, on Facebook at facebook.com/totalhealthnutrition, and on Twitter at @healthrd.

Printed in the USA
CPSIA information can be obtained
at www.ICGtesting.com
CBHW040738280124
3678CB00002B/16